Pathology

PRETEST Self-Assessment and Review

Edited by
Ronald Daniel Neumann, M.D.
Yale-New Haven Medical Center
New Haven, Connecticut

Basic Sciences:
PreTest Self-Assessment and Review Series

John Watkins Foster, Jr., M.D., Editor
Yale-New Haven Medical Center
New Haven, Connecticut

Robert Edwards Humphreys, M.D., Ph.D., Editor
University of Massachusetts Medical School
Worcester, Massachusetts

PreTest Service, Inc.,

Distributed by Blakiston Publications
McGraw-Hill Book Company

© 1976 by PreTest Service, Inc. All rights reserved. Printed in the United States of America. No part of this publication may be reproduced, stored in a retrieval system, or transmitted, in any form or by any means, electronic, mechanical, photocopying, recording, or otherwise, without the prior written permission of the publisher.

Library of Congress Catalog Card Number: 76-2598

ISBN: 0-07-050794-5

Editor: Mary Ann C. Sheldon
Typographer: Elaine Reid
Production Staff: Donna D' Amico, Pamela G. Oliano, Judith M. Raccio
Layout: Robert Tutsky
Illustrator: Leonard Galushko
Cover Design: Silverman Design
Printer: Connecticut Printers

NOTICE

Medicine is an ever-changing science. As new research and clinical experience broaden our knowledge, changes in treatment and drug therapy are required. The editors and the publisher of this work have made every effort to ensure that the drug dosage schedules herein are accurate and in accord with the standards accepted at the time of publication. Readers are advised, however, to check the product information sheet included in the package of each drug they plan to administer to be certain that changes have not been made in the recommended dose or in the contraindications for administration. This recommendation is of particular importance in regard to new or infrequently used drugs.

PRINT NUMBER: 9   8   7   6   5   4   3   2

Contents

List of Contributors iv

Part One: Questions

General Pathology 1
Hematology 23
Cardiovascular System 39
Respiratory System 49
Gastrointestinal System 57
Endocrine System 69
Genitourinary System 74
Nervous System 90
Skeletomuscular System 97
Skin and Breast 107

Part Two: Answers, Explanations, and References

General Pathology 117
Hematology 135
Cardiovascular System 142
Respiratory System 148
Gastrointestinal System 152
Endocrine System 157
Genitourinary System 161
Nervous System 170
Skeletomuscular System 177
Skin and Breast 182

Bibliography 187

List of Contributors

Jane Barry, M.D.
Yale-New Haven Medical Center
New Haven, Connecticut

Stewart Fox, M.D.
Yale-New Haven Medical Center
New Haven, Connecticut

Stephen Gray, M.D.
U. S. Army Hospital
Landstuhl, West Germany

Donald Francis Haggerty, Ph.D.
University of California, Los Angeles
Los Angeles, California

T. Ralph Hollands, M.D., Ph.D.
McMaster University
Hamilton, Ontario, Canada

John T. Homer, Ph.D.
University of Oklahoma
Stillwater, Oklahoma

Thomas Johnson, M.D.
Yale-New Haven Medical Center
New Haven, Connecticut

L. James Kennedy, Jr., M.D.
University of Colorado,
School of Medicine
Denver, Colorado

John Kirkwood, M.D.
Yale-New Haven Medical Center
New Haven, Connecticut

John Kozarich, Ph.D.
Harvard University
Cambridge, Massachusetts

Ian Love, M.D.
Yale-New Haven Medical Center
New Haven, Connecticut

Lore Ann McNicol, Ph.D.
University of Pennsylvania
School of Medicine
Philadelphia, Pennsylvania

Monique Minor, M.D.
Yale-New Haven Medical Center
New Haven, Connecticut

Ronald Daniel Neumann, M.D.
Yale-New Haven Medical Center
New Haven, Connecticut

David A. Pearson, Ph.D.
Yale-New Haven Medical Center
New Haven, Connecticut

Duane L. Peavy, Ph.D.
Harvard Medical School
Boston, Massachusetts

Mary Lake Polan, M.D., Ph.D.
Yale-New Haven Medical Center
New Haven, Connecticut

William Schoene, M.D.
Harvard Medical School
Boston, Massachusetts

Richard Staimen, M.D.
Fort Devens Army Hospital
Ayre, Massachusetts

Daniel Carl Sullivan, M.D.
Yale-New Haven Medical Center
New Haven, Connecticut

Gary Boyd Thurman, Ph.D.
University of Texas Medical Branch
Galveston, Texas

Prabhakar Narhari Vaidya, M.D.
Oak Forest Hospital
Oak Forest, Illinois

Richard Weiss, Ph.D.
University of California
Irvine, California

Stephen White, Ph.D.
University of Chicago
Chicago, Illinois

General Pathology

DIRECTIONS: Each question below contains five suggested answers. Choose the **one best** response to each question.

1. An increase in tissue volume without addition of new cells is

(A) anaplasia
(B) hyperplasia
(C) hypertrophy
(D) metaplasia
(E) neoplasia

2. A heart which is abnormally large but does not have an increase in the number of cells is

(A) atrophied
(B) hypertrophied
(C) dysplastic
(D) hyperplastic
(E) anaplastic

3. Which of the following has the greatest regenerative capacity?

(A) Myocardium
(B) Cartilage
(C) Connective tissue
(D) Voluntary muscle
(E) Central nervous system neurons

4. The type of cell that is first to migrate into foci of acute inflammation is the

(A) plasma cell
(B) polymorphonuclear leukocyte
(C) lymphocyte
(D) monocyte
(E) fibroblast

5. Metaplasia is

(A) a change in which one adult cell type is replaced by another adult cell type
(B) always premalignant
(C) extreme hyperplasia
(D) extreme hypoplasia
(E) shrinkage in the size of a cell

6. Chronic inflammations most often contain

(A) eosinophils
(B) neutrophils
(C) basophils
(D) lymphocytes
(E) endothelial cells

7. Catarrhal inflammation is characterized by

(A) deep ulceration
(B) discharge from superficial mucosal surfaces
(C) abscess formation
(D) cellulitis
(E) granulomatous reaction

8. Which of the following organs is most severely affected by shock?

(A) Liver
(B) Lung
(C) Heart
(D) Kidney
(E) Adrenal gland

9. The cluster of cells in the photograph below appeared in a cytologic specimen of sputum from a 57-year-old man with chest pain, hemoptysis, and a nonproductive cough of many years' duration. What is the most likely diagnosis?

(A) Squamous cell metaplasia of ciliated, bronchial epithelium
(B) Oat cell (small cell undifferentiated) carcinoma
(C) Adenocarcinoma
(D) Cytomegalic inclusion virus pneumonia
(E) Normal bronchial epithelium

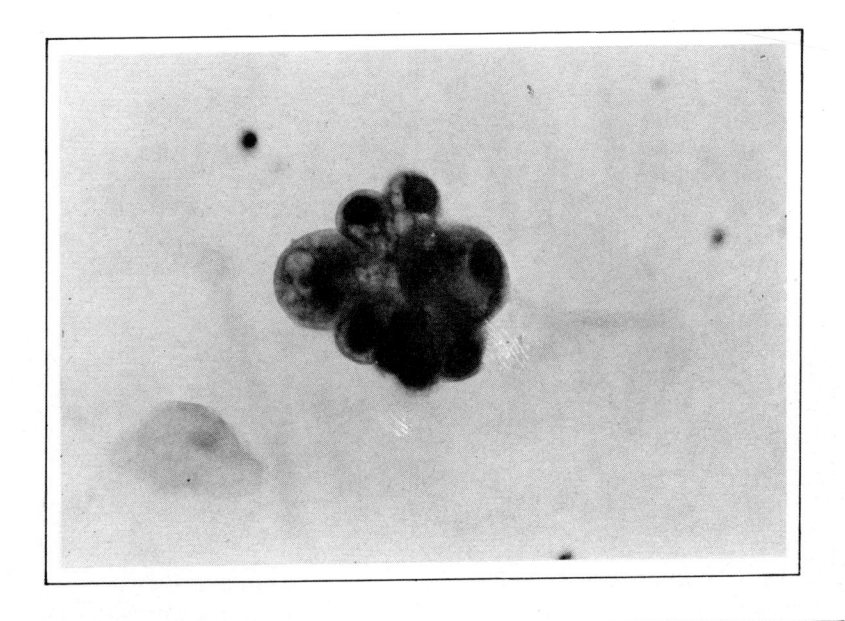

10. Which of the following types of tumors is the most sensitive to radiation?

(A) Malignant lymphoma
(B) Basal cell carcinoma
(C) Cervical carcinoma
(D) Osteogenic sarcoma
(E) Malignant melanoma

11. The most common malignancy of the oral cavity is

(A) adenocarcinoma
(B) squamous cell carcinoma
(C) malignant melanoma
(D) fibrosarcoma
(E) lymphosarcoma

12. The cells in the photograph shown below are from a drop of cerebrospinal fluid. The most likely diagnosis is

(A) subarachnoid hemorrhage
(B) viral meningitis
(C) tuberculous meningitis
(D) bacterial meningitis
(E) leukemic meningitis

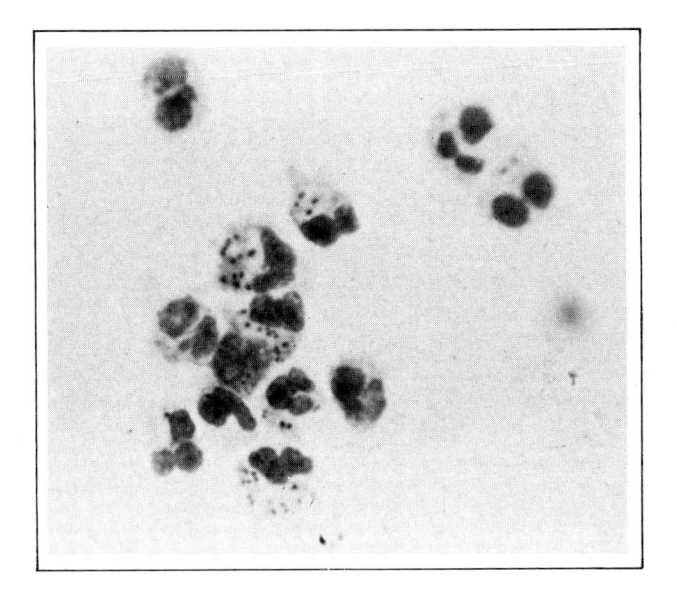

13. Sarcomas characteristically metastasize

(A) as emboli in the lymphatic system
(B) by direct growth along lymphatic channels
(C) as emboli in the bloodstream
(D) by direct growth along blood vessels
(E) by detachment and reimplantation in body cavities

14. Carcinomas commonly metastasize to all of the following sites EXCEPT

(A) lung
(B) liver
(C) kidney
(D) skeletal muscle
(E) lymph nodes

15. The eggs shown in the photograph below were obtained from the perianal region of a child by scotch tape swab. The infecting organism is

(A) *Enterobius vermicularis*
(B) *Trichuris trichiura*
(C) *Ancylostoma duodenale*
(D) *Taenia saginata*
(E) *Schistosoma haematobium*

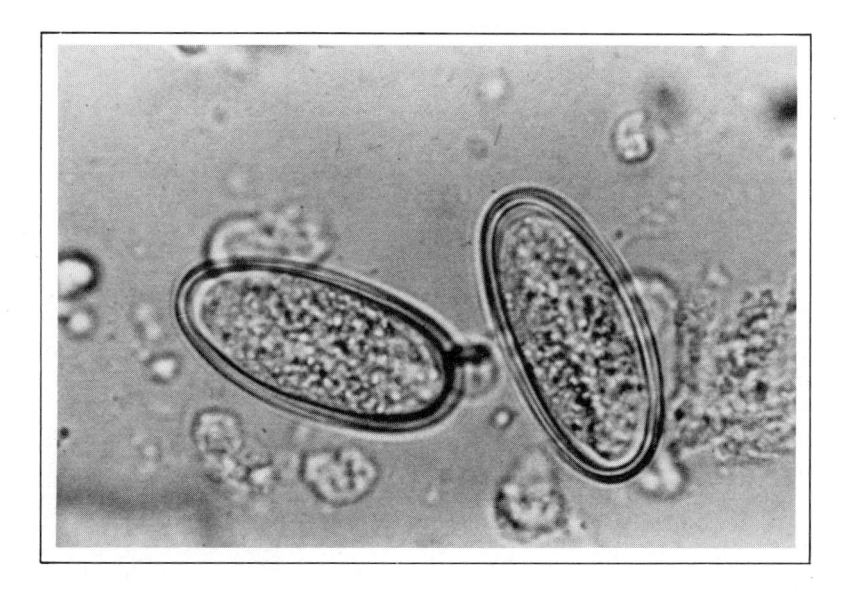

16. The lymph node shown on the facing page was probably excised from a patient with

(A) sickle cell anemia
(B) carcinoma
(C) leukemia
(D) infectious mononucleosis
(E) rheumatoid arthritis

17. The lesion in the photograph shown on the facing page was removed from a discrete mass in the retroperitoneum. It is a

(A) lymphoma
(B) neuroma
(C) fibroma
(D) fibrosarcoma
(E) carcinoma

Photograph accompanies Question 16

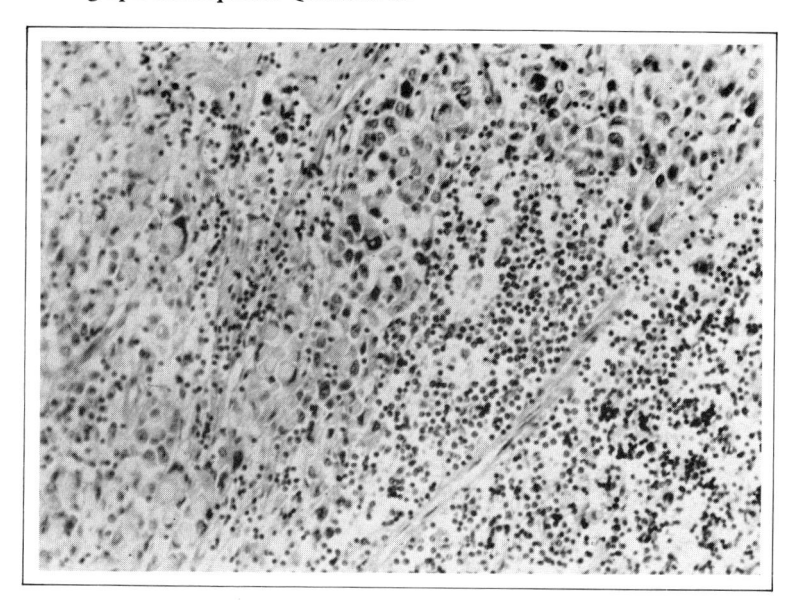

Photograph accompanies Question 17

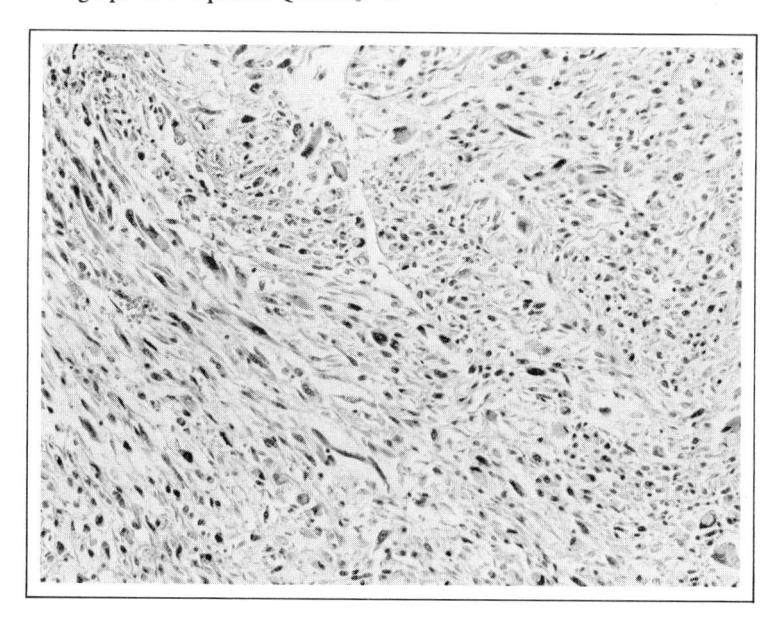

18. The irregular eosinophilic hyaline inclusions within the hepatocyte cytoplasm shown below are

(A) Russell bodies
(B) characteristic of alcoholism
(C) associated with viral hepatitis
(D) secondary to carbon tetrachloride poisoning
(E) parasites

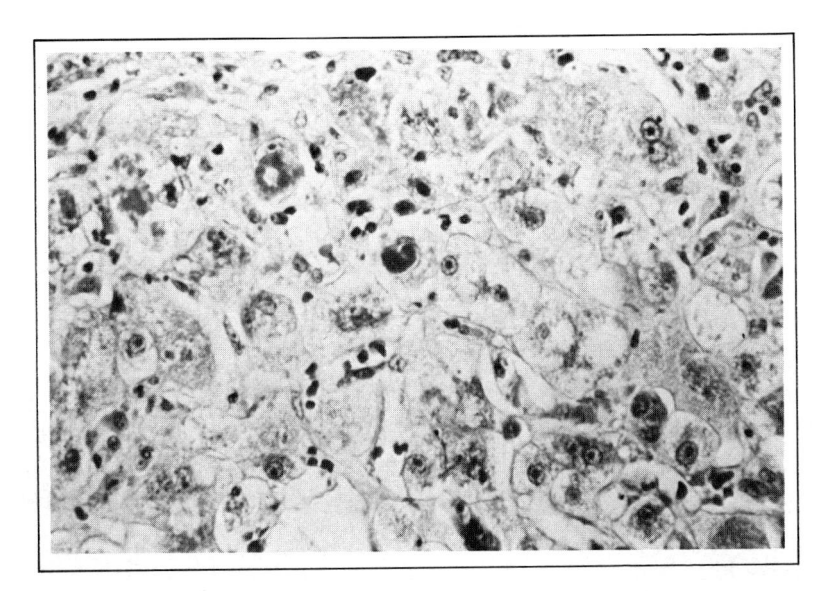

19. Niemann-Pick disease is characterized by

(A) the accumulation of sphingomyelin
(B) the accumulation of gangliosides
(C) the accumulation of kerasin
(D) diabetes insipidus
(E) nonlipid reticuloendotheliosis

20. The diseases of the Hand-Schüller-Christian complex all involve the

(A) skeleton
(B) reticuloendothelial system
(C) heart
(D) lungs
(E) teeth and nails

21. All of the following symptoms are associated with Klinefelter's syndrome EXCEPT

(A) large, soft testes
(B) gynecomastia
(C) clumping of Leydig cells
(D) azospermia
(E) elevated urinary gonadotropins

22. Which of the following is NOT a manifestation of the Laurence-Moon-Biedl syndrome?

(A) Dolichocephaly
(B) Mental retardation
(C) Obesity
(D) Retinitis pigmentosa
(E) Polydactyly

23. Leukocytes deficient in oxidase activity, inability to destroy staphylococcal bacteria, and recurrent infections beginning in the first year of life are characteristic of

(A) chronic granulomatous disease
(B) congenital agammaglobulinemia
(C) hereditary thymic dysplasia
(D) Chédiak-Higashi syndrome
(E) Wiskott-Aldrich syndrome

24. Pellagra is a clinical deficiency syndrome resulting from a lack of

(A) pantothenic acid
(B) cyanocobalamine
(C) riboflavin
(D) nicotinamide
(E) pyridoxine

25. Mumps, Mikulicz syndrome, and alcoholic pancreatitis may all be associated with an elevated serum level of

(A) amylase
(B) serum glutamic-oxaloacetic transaminase (SGOT)
(C) lactic dehydrogenase (LDH)
(D) bilirubin
(E) ammonia

26. Blindness and metabolic acidosis are common findings in poisoning caused by

(A) carbon monoxide
(B) benzene
(C) phenol
(D) chloroform
(E) methyl alcohol

27. Fibrinoid contains

(A) immunoglobulins
(B) fat
(C) hemosiderin
(D) glycogen
(E) amyloid

28. Wilson's disease results from the deposition of copper in the tissues. The increased copper is localized primarily in the liver, brain, kidneys, and

(A) skin
(B) hair
(C) bone
(D) tooth enamel
(E) cornea

29. Ochronosis, as a congenital metabolic disorder, is associated with an excessive accumulation of homogentisic acid in the

(A) cartilage
(B) dermis of the skin
(C) large bowel mucosa
(D) medullary cavity of the long bones
(E) white matter of the brain

30. Gout is thought to result from a disturbance in the metabolism of

(A) pyrimidine
(B) folate
(C) histone
(D) purine
(E) lipid

31. The cell shown in the photograph below is an example of

(A) erythrophagocytosis
(B) tart cells
(C) lupus erythematosus (LE) cells
(D) atypical lymphocytes
(E) staining artifacts

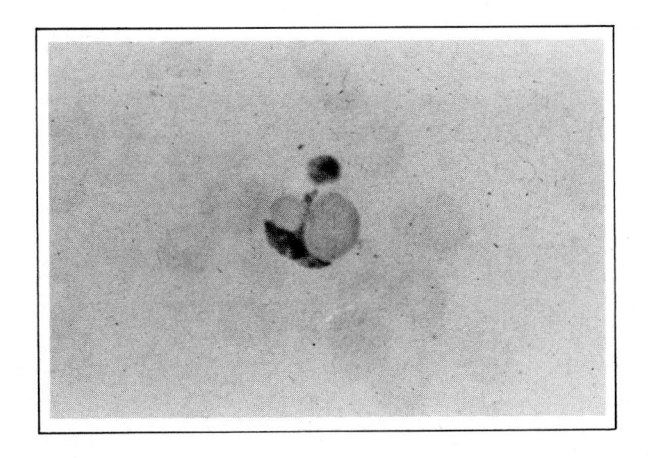

32. The absence of the enzyme glucose 6-phosphatase in liver and kidney cells is characteristic of

(A) von Gierke's disease
(B) McArdle's disease
(C) Pompe's disease
(D) Crigler-Najjar syndrome
(E) Gilbert syndrome

33. An allograft is a graft between

(A) a man and an animal
(B) two individuals of different species
(C) two individuals of the same species
(D) two individuals of the same inbred strain
(E) identical twins

34. Which of the following conditions is most likely to be associated with cancer?

(A) Systemic lupus erythematosus
(B) Hypertension
(C) Polymyositis
(D) Autoimmune thyroiditis
(E) Arteriosclerosis

35. In systemic lupus erythematosus which of the following findings has the highest correlation with morbidity and mortality?

(A) LE cells
(B) Lupus nephritis
(C) Lupus endocarditis
(D) Thrombocytopenia
(E) Skin lesions

36. The presence of high titers of antibodies to the nuclear proteins of multiple different tissue types is characteristic of

(A) leukemia
(B) lupus erythematosus
(C) periarteritis nodosa
(D) chronic active hepatitis
(E) poststreptococcal glomerulonephritis

37. Tangier disease is a rare disorder characterized by almost complete absence of plasma

(A) glyceride
(B) cholesterol
(C) high-density lipoprotein
(D) low-density lipoprotein
(E) sphingosine

38. A common feature of xanthinuria is the almost total replacement by xanthine of urinary

(A) hypoxanthine
(B) guanine
(C) orotic acid
(D) uric acid
(E) 7-methyl-8-hydroxyguanine

39. The subnormal serum alkaline phosphatase activity in the familial disease hypophosphatasia offers strong support for a role of this enzyme in

(A) calcification of bone
(B) nucleotide synthesis
(C) heme biosynthesis
(D) skeletal muscle development
(E) loss of hair

40. The most specific immunologic test for diagnosing primary biliary cirrhosis is a test for the presence of

(A) antimitochondrial antibodies
(B) antinuclear antibodies
(C) antiplatelet antibodies
(D) smooth muscle antibodies
(E) Dane particles

41. Rheumatoid factor is an antibody which reacts most strongly with

(A) immunoglobulin A
(B) immunoglobulin G
(C) immunoglobulin M
(D) joint synovial membrane
(E) inorganic crystaloids

42. Normal levels of C-reactive protein (CRP) are most often observed in

(A) acute viral illness
(B) pneumococcal pneumonia
(C) active rheumatoid arthritis
(D) pulmonary tuberculosis
(E) acute myocardial infarct

43. The most sensitive of the commonly used tests for diagnosing active syphilis is the

(A) rapid plasma reagin test (RPR)
(B) *Treponema pallidum* immobilization test (TPI)
(C) fluorescent treponemal antibody-absorption test (FTA-ABS)
(D) Venereal Disease Research Laboratory test (VDRL)
(E) Kolmer test

44. Features commonly seen in tuberculoid leprosy include all the following EXCEPT the

(A) presence of large numbers of bacilli in involved tissues
(B) extension of chronic plasmacytic and lymphocytic infiltrates into the papillary dermis
(C) severe infiltration of small nerves by chronic inflammatory cells
(D) destruction of nerves early in the course of the disease
(E) proliferation of epithelioid cells which are arranged in clusters and cords

45. In granuloma inguinale, the causative microbe, *Donovania granulomatis*, can most often be demonstrated within

(A) neutrophils
(B) eosinophils
(C) lymphocytes
(D) monocytes
(E) plasma cells

46. Spirochetal infections include all of the following EXCEPT

(A) bejel
(B) yaws
(C) pinta
(D) Weil's disease
(E) lymphogranuloma venereum

47. The presence of an elevated cerebrospinal fluid IgG level and an abnormal band on agar gel electrophoresis of the CSF is consistent with the diagnosis of

(A) secondary stage of syphilis
(B) muscular dystrophy
(C) tumor involvement of the spinal cord
(D) meningeal involvement by leukemia
(E) multiple sclerosis

48. Which of the following conditions is most likely to give a *"negative"* result on routine pregnancy tests?

(A) Ectopic pregnancy
(B) Hydatidiform mole
(C) Polyhydramnios
(D) Eclampsia
(E) Choriocarcinoma

49. An infant with a sweat chloride value of 80 mEq/l (normal = <50 mEq/l) is likely to have

(A) diabetes mellitus
(B) hypoadrenalism
(C) dermatomyositis
(D) cystic fibrosis
(E) scleroderma

50. A fasting blood sample reveals a clear serum, a normal level of serum triglyceride, and a serum cholesterol level of 975 mg/100 ml (normal = <300 mg/100 ml). These findings are consistent with hyperlipoproteinemia of which of the following types?

(A) Type I
(B) Type II
(C) Type III
(D) Type IV
(E) Type V

51. Which curve in the figure shown below represents a "normal" glucose tolerance test?

(A) A
(B) B
(C) C
(D) D
(E) E

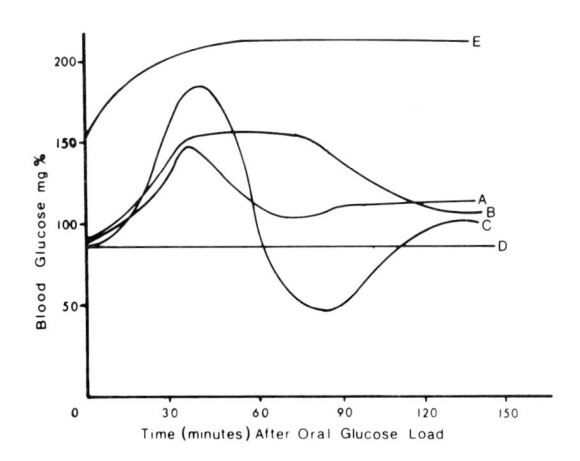

52. The enzyme activity curve shown below best represents the pattern for which serum enzyme after an uncomplicated acute myocardial infarct?

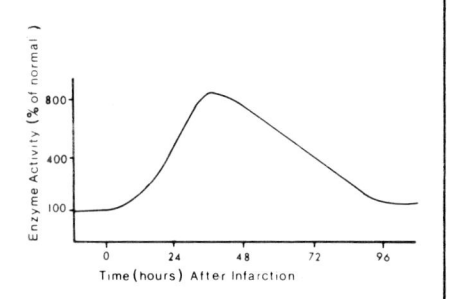

(A) Serum glutamic-oxaloacetic transaminase (SGOT)
(B) Creatinine phosphokinase (CPK)
(C) Lactic dehydrogenase (LDH)
(D) Alkaline phosphatase
(E) 5′-Nucleotidase

53. Parathyroid hormone does NOT cause

(A) increased intestinal calcium absorption
(B) increased renal absorption of calcium
(C) mobilization of calcium from bone
(D) increased plasma phosphate levels
(E) decreased renal absorption of phosphate

54. Consider the following electrolyte values: pH 7.58; sodium 140 mEq/l; chloride 80 mEq/l; potassium 3.9 mEq/l; and total CO_2 content 48 mmol/l. They are compatible with

(A) severe diabetes mellitus
(B) aspirin ingestion
(C) severe vomiting
(D) hepatic coma
(E) shock

55. Parkinsonism is associated with

(A) arbovirus encephalitis
(B) encephalitis lethargica (Economo's disease)
(C) St. Louis encephalitis
(D) equine encephalitis
(E) lymphocytic choriomeningitis

56. The most comprehensive determination of adrenocortical function can be obtained by measurement of

(A) urinary 17-hydroxysteroids
(B) urinary 17-ketosteroids
(C) urinary 17-ketogenic steroids
(D) plasma cortisol
(E) plasma aldosterone

57. A lower than normal serum amylase level may be seen in patients who have

(A) diabetes mellitus
(B) an overdose of narcotic analgesics
(C) mumps
(D) renal insufficiency
(E) a ruptured ectopic pregnancy

58. What is the creatinine clearance of a person who passes 361 mg of creatinine in a 24-hour urine sample of 770 ml, and whose serum creatinine is 2.0 mg/100 ml?

(A) 12.5 ml/min
(B) 25.0 ml/min
(C) 50.0 ml/min
(D) 75.0 ml/min
(E) 100 ml/min

59. Which of the following would be contraindicated in an individual with hyperuricemia?

(A) Large amounts of citrus fruit
(B) Large volumes of cranberry juice
(C) A diet low in meat
(D) Large doses of salicylates
(E) Allopurinol

60. Bence Jones proteins found in urine or in serum represent

(A) cryoglobulins
(B) immunoglobulin light chains
(C) immunoglobulin heavy chains
(D) amyloid
(E) cell wall proteins of *Mycoplasma pneumoniae*

61. Which of the following proteins is NOT observed in a serum immunoelectrophoresis performed on cellulose acetate at pH 8.6?

(A) α_2-Macroglobulin
(B) Albumin
(C) α_1-Antitrypsin
(D) IgM
(E) Fibrinogen

62. An elevation of serum acid phosphatase may be found in

(A) ulcerative colitis
(B) hepatocellular carcinoma
(C) diabetes mellitus
(D) polycythemia vera
(E) chronic cholangitis

63. Graves' disease is associated with elevated levels of

(A) long-acting thyroid stimulator (LATS)
(B) thyroid-stimulating hormone (TSH)
(C) adrenocorticotropic hormone (ACTH)
(D) human chorionic gonadotropin (HCG)
(E) growth hormone (GH)

64. The section of lung in the photograph below was stained with a silver-containing stain. It reveals the presence of

65. The diagram below shows the normal serum values for the five isozymes of lactic dehydrogenase (LDH) and the values obtained for one patient. The diagnosis most compatible with the patient's values is

Isozyme	Normal % activity	Patient's % activity
LDH_1	20–35	18
LDH_2	30–40	24
LDH_3	20–30	13
LDH_4	5–15	26
LDH_5	1–15	19

(A) acute hepatitis
(B) pernicious anemia
(C) pulmonary infarct
(D) myocardial infarct
(E) cerebrovascular accident

(A) fungi
(B) asbestos particles
(C) *Mycobacterium tuberculosis*
(D) *Pneumocystis carinii*
(E) bronchiolitis obliterans

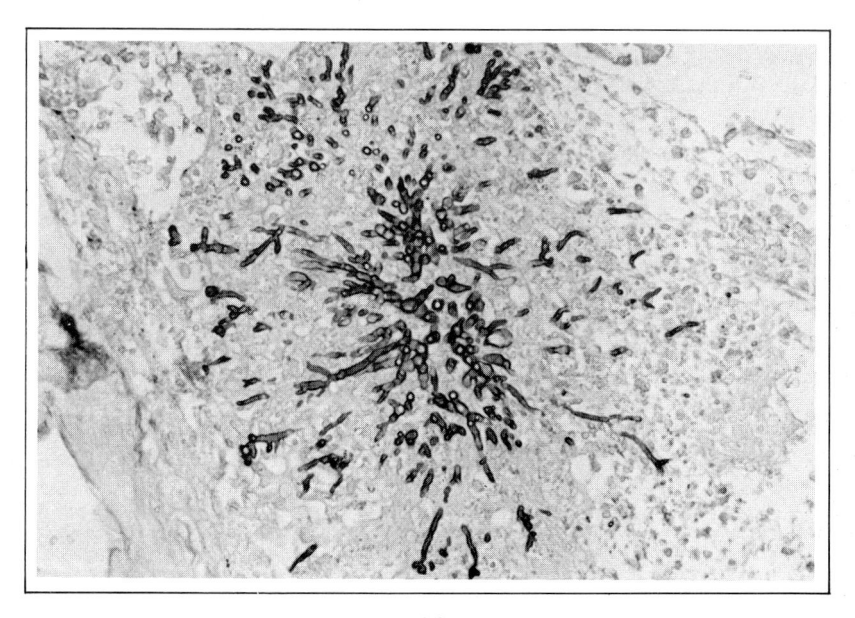

66. Which of the following statements is NOT true of fungi of the order Mucorales?

(A) They are fungi of low virulence
(B) They are encountered clinically most often in debilitated patients
(C) They can be recognized by their septate hyphae
(D) They are readily stained by the periodic acid-Schiff (PAS) technique
(E) They are most often encountered in lungs, hairy paranasal sinuses, and the middle ear

67. Which of the following is physiologically the most active thyroid hormone?

(A) Thyroglobulin
(B) Monoiodotyrosine (MIT)
(C) Diiodotyrosine (DIT)
(D) Triiodothyronine (T_3)
(E) Thyroxine (T_4)

68. Most patients with primary hemochromatosis become symptomatic between the ages of

(A) 1 and 4 weeks
(B) 1 and 3 years
(C) 3 and 7 years
(D) 10 and 20 years
(E) 40 and 60 years

69. Primary gout is a genetic disorder of purine metabolism in which the main biochemical feature is

(A) excessive excretion of uric acid
(B) excessive excretion of xanthine
(C) excessive excretion of orotic acid
(D) hyperuricemia
(E) hypouricemia

70. Certain types of congenital virilizing adrenocortical hyperplasia result in

(A) calcium deposits similar to oxalosis
(B) accumulation of glycolipids in tissues
(C) salt loss simulating Addison's disease
(D) symptoms similar to phenylketonuria
(E) severe acidosis

71. In Tay-Sachs disease, over 90 percent of the accumulated gangliosides are lacking

(A) sphingosine
(B) the terminal galactose
(C) the fatty acid moiety
(D) a hexosamine moiety
(E) the entire carbohydrate moiety

72. The severity of most cases of pentosuria is usually

(A) variable
(B) asymptomatic except for accidental circumstance
(C) mild to moderate
(D) severe to lethal
(E) asymptomatic and without consequence

73. Renal tubular acidosis is characterized by

(A) a low concentration of serum bicarbonate and an approximately commensurate elevation in serum chloride
(B) a low concentration of serum chloride and an approximately commensurate elevation in serum bicarbonate
(C) low concentrations of both serum chloride and bicarbonate
(D) high concentrations of both serum chloride and bicarbonate
(E) high serum potassium levels

74. The major underlying defect in renal tubular acidosis appears to be

(A) an excessive back-diffusion of secreted hydrogen from tubular urine to blood
(B) an impairment of ammonia excretion
(C) a leakage of bicarbonate out of the proximal tubule
(D) a deficiency in the total hydrogen secretory capacity
(E) an impairment in the reclamation of filtered bicarbonate

75. Which of the following disorders of porphyrin metabolism is NOT associated with cutaneous sensitivity?

(A) Erythropoietic porphyria
(B) Congenital erythropoietic porphyria
(C) Variegata porphyria
(D) Intermittent acute porphyria
(E) Günther's disease

76. Nonpathogenic pneumococci typically exhibit

(A) R (rough) genotypes
(B) positive quellung reactions
(C) alpha-hemolysis when grown on blood agar
(D) bile-solubility when grown in deoxycholate media
(E) positive reactions on exposure to type 3 antisera

77. Which of the following bacteria is an immobile gram-negative rod that grows in large mucoid colonies, can synthesize butylene glycol but not indole, and is incapable of decarboxylating ornithine?

(A) *Escherichia coli*
(B) *Salmonella typhosa*
(C) *Klebsiella pneumoniae*
(D) *Proteus vulgaris*
(E) *Proteus mirabilis*

78. Characteristically, T lymphocytes do NOT

(A) affect cell-mediated immunity
(B) occur as the most common lymphocyte of peripheral blood
(C) secrete immunoglobulin G
(D) occur in the interfollicular portion of lymph nodes
(E) contain the theta surface antigen

79. Which immunoglobulin plays the dominant role in immunity for the mucosal surfaces of the respiratory and gastrointestinal tract?

(A) IgA
(B) IgD
(C) IgE
(D) IgG
(E) IgM

80. Antibody deposition on basement membrane is characteristic of

(A) rheumatoid arthritis
(B) Hashimoto's disease
(C) primary biliary cirrhosis
(D) pernicious anemia
(E) Goodpasture's syndrome

81. Delayed-type hypersensitivity reactions of the tuberculin skin test type

(A) appear within one or two hours
(B) require an intact T lymphocyte population
(C) show dermal infiltrates of granulocytes
(D) are associated uniquely with small antigens
(E) do not require previous exposure to the antigen

82. Large amounts of antigen are required to produce

(A) serum sickness
(B) an Arthus reaction
(C) generalized anaphylaxis
(D) cutaneous anaphylaxis
(E) atopic responses

83. Bacteriophage-mediated alteration of bacterial genetic pools is called

(A) conjugation
(B) recombination
(C) transduction
(D) transcription
(E) transformation

84. Picornaviruses can cause all of the following EXCEPT

(A) the "common cold"
(B) poliomyelitis
(C) keratoconjunctivitis
(D) aseptic meningitis
(E) herpangina

85. Under aerobic conditions, which of the following organisms will NOT grow on heat-treated chocolate agar unless another organism such as *Staphylococcus aureus* is growing in its vicinity?

(A) *Bordetella bronchiseptica*
(B) *Bordetella pertussis*
(C) *Hemophilus ducreyi*
(D) *Hemophilus influenzae*
(E) *Diplococcus pneumoniae*

86. All of the following statements about *Mycobacterium tuberculosis* are true EXCEPT

(A) it has a long doubling time
(B) its cell wall contains large amounts of lipid
(C) it is associated with silica miners
(D) it is prone to drug-resistant mutation
(E) it is a facultative anaerobe

87. Which of the following organisms is highly pathogenic in humans, grows as an encapsulated yeast both in culture and in infected tissues, and often produces a chronic, exudative meningitis?

(A) *Aspergillus fumigatus*
(B) *Histoplasma capsulatum*
(C) *Coccidioides immitis*
(D) *Cryptococcus neoformans*
(E) *Blastomyces dermatitidis*

88. Which of the following diseases is NOT associated with herpesviruses?

(A) Mononucleosis
(B) Shingles
(C) Influenza
(D) Cytomegalic inclusion disease
(E) Chickenpox (varicella)

89. The presence in the serum of cold-reacting antibodies, as well as antibodies against specific alpha-hemolytic streptococci, is compatible with the diagnosis of

(A) *Mycoplasma pneumoniae*
(B) *Diplococcus pneumoniae*
(C) *Nocardia asteroides*
(D) Influenza virus
(E) Cytomegalovirus

90. Exotoxins are NOT produced by

(A) *Salmonella typhi*
(B) *Bordetella pertussis*
(C) *Staphylococcus aureus*
(D) *Corynebacterium diphtheriae*
(E) *Clostridium tetani*

91. Abscess formation is commonly associated with

(A) primary atypical pneumonia
(B) staphylococcal pneumonia
(C) lobar pneumonia
(D) *Klebsiella pneumoniae*
(E) asbestosis

92. The hepatic microabscess shown below was one of many found on autopsy, in the liver, lungs, and adrenal glands of a 5-day-old male infant with a concomitant vesicular skin eruption. The lesion shown by the arrow is most consistent with infection by a

(A) virus
(B) yeast
(C) bacterial coccal form
(D) helminth
(E) protozoa

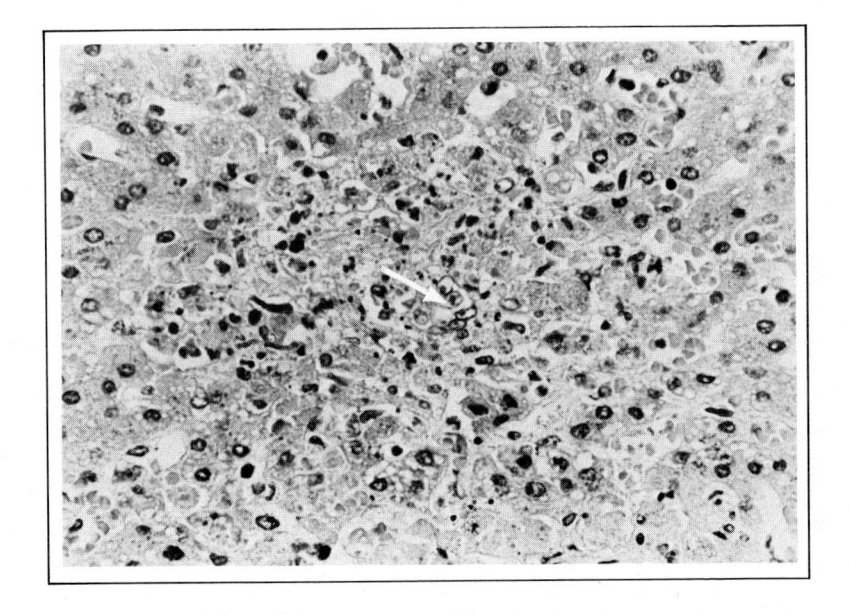

DIRECTIONS: Each question below contains four suggested answers of which **one** or **more** is correct. Choose the answer

A	if	1, 2, and 3	are correct
B	if	1 and 3	are correct
C	if	2 and 4	are correct
D	if	4	is correct
E	if	1, 2, 3, and 4	are correct

93. Coagulation necrosis is seen in

(1) ischemic infarction
(2) gummas
(3) mercurial poisoning
(4) Zenker's hyaline degeneration

94. Dystrophic calcification

(1) occurs in dead or dying tissue
(2) occurs in healthy tissue
(3) may occur in the presence of normal serum calcium
(4) almost always reflects some abnormality of calcium metabolism

95. Mononuclear phagocytes of the reticuloendothelial system include

(1) Kupffer cells
(2) Langhans' giant cells
(3) heart-failure cells
(4) plasma cells

96. Radiosensitive tissues that can be damaged or killed by doses of 2500 R or less include

(1) kidney
(2) liver
(3) skeletal muscle cells
(4) intestinal epithelium

97. Inflammation of adipose tissue is a common morphologic feature of

(1) intestinal lipodystrophy
(2) insulin lipodystrophy
(3) sclerema neonatorum
(4) steatopygia

98. Fat necrosis occurs in

(1) acute pancreatitis
(2) hyperlipidemia
(3) traumatized breast tissue
(4) hibernomas

99. Secondary gout may be seen in association with

(1) polycythemia
(2) psoriasis
(3) hemolytic anemias
(4) myeloproliferative diseases

100. The plaques of atherosclerosis are located mainly

(1) under the basement membrane
(2) within the media
(3) within the adventitia
(4) within the intima

101. Increased deposition of hemosiderin, as shown below in a liver section stained with Prussian blue, may

(1) result from excessive dietary intake
(2) be associated with bronze diabetes
(3) occur in pulmonary macrophages in chronic heart failure
(4) be associated with cirrhosis

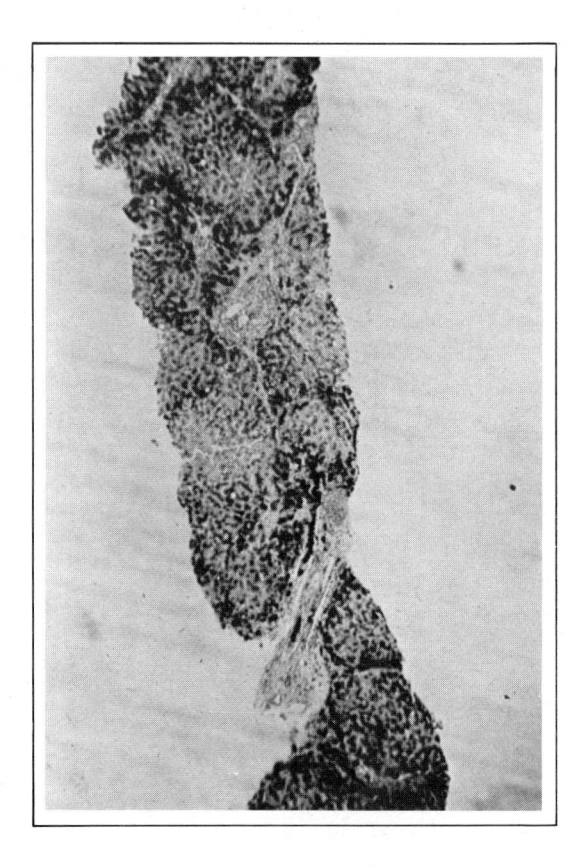

102. Vitamin D deficiency might be expected to lead to a

(1) relative excess of osteoid tissue in bone
(2) decreased production of bone matrix
(3) decreased absorption of calcium
(4) reduced collagen formation

103. Which of the following diseases are glycogen storage diseases?

(1) Von Gierke's disease
(2) Pompe's disease
(3) McArdle's disease
(4) Tay-Sachs disease

SUMMARY OF DIRECTIONS				
A	B	C	D	E
1, 2, 3 only	1, 3 only	2, 4 only	4 only	All are correct

104. Morphologic alterations observed in women taking oral contraceptives include

(1) formation of ovarian follicular cysts
(2) intimal fibrosis and endothelial proliferation in small pulmonary arteries
(3) deep vein thrombosis
(4) hepatocellular necrosis and bile duct hyperplasia

105. Vitamins that are toxic if ingested in excessive quantities include

(1) thiamine (B_1)
(2) vitamin A
(3) ascorbic acid (C)
(4) vitamin D

106. Diffuse scleroderma (progressive systemic sclerosis) is characterized by

(1) depression of gamma globulin in a majority of patients
(2) degeneration of collagen
(3) higher incidence in men than women
(4) involvement of the gastrointestinal tract

107. Which of the following occur with a plasmacytoma?

(1) Bence Jones proteinuria
(2) Gamma-Gandy bodies
(3) Abnormal serum globulins
(4) Massive pulmonary emboli

108. Rickettsial diseases include

(1) typhus
(2) trench fever
(3) Q fever
(4) trachoma

109. Viruses that produce intracellular inclusions in tissue sections include

(1) measles virus
(2) adenovirus
(3) cytomegalovirus
(4) varicella virus

110. The Epstein-Barr (EB) virus is associated with

(1) infectious mononucleosis
(2) nasopharyngeal carcinoma
(3) Burkitt's lymphoma
(4) cat-scratch fever

111. Which of the following diseases are characterized by granulomatous lesions?

(1) Tularemia
(2) Lymphogranuloma inguinale
(3) Brucellosis
(4) Glanders

112. Which of the following observations support the contention that host immunity plays a role in cancer?

(1) The increased incidence of cancer in immunosuppressed allograft recipients
(2) The presence of "blocking antibodies" in patients with cancer
(3) The presence of tumor-specific antibodies in patients with cancer
(4) The presence of anergy in patients with cancer

DIRECTIONS: The groups of questions in this section consist of five lettered headings followed by several numbered items. For each numbered item choose the **one** lettered heading with which it is **most** closely associated. Each lettered heading may be used once, more than once, or not at all.

Questions 113-115
For each tumor, choose its diagnostic serum protein.

(A) Acid phosphatase
(B) Carcinoembryonic antigen
(C) α_1-Fetoprotein
(D) β-Fetoprotein
(E) β_2-Microglobulin

113. Hepatoma

114. Gastrointestinal carcinoma

115. Prostatic carcinoma

Questions 116-119
For each clinical situation, choose the immune agent responsible.

(A) T-Lymphocytes
(B) IgA
(C) IgD
(D) IgE
(E) IgM

116. Tuberculin reaction

117. Allograft rejection

118. Hay fever

119. Anaphylaxis

Questions 120-123
For each immunoglobulin, choose the characteristic with which it is most likely to be associated.

(A) Cytophilic for mast cells
(B) Secretory piece
(C) Appears first in a primary immune response
(D) Constitutes 80 percent of the circulating gamma globulin in adults
(E) A component of HL-A histocompatibility antigen

120. IgG

121. IgM

122. IgA

123. IgE

Hematology

DIRECTIONS: Each question below contains five suggested answers. Choose the **one best** response to each question.

124. Early signs of a serious hemolytic reaction to a mismatched blood transfusion may include all of the following EXCEPT

(A) excessive oozing at the operative site
(B) restlessness
(C) anxiety
(D) precordial pain
(E) bradycardia

125. The pink-staining structure seen below in the cytoplasm of an immature leukocyte is

(A) a platelet
(B) a Howell-Jolly body
(C) an Auer body
(D) a Pappenheimer body
(E) a Döhle body

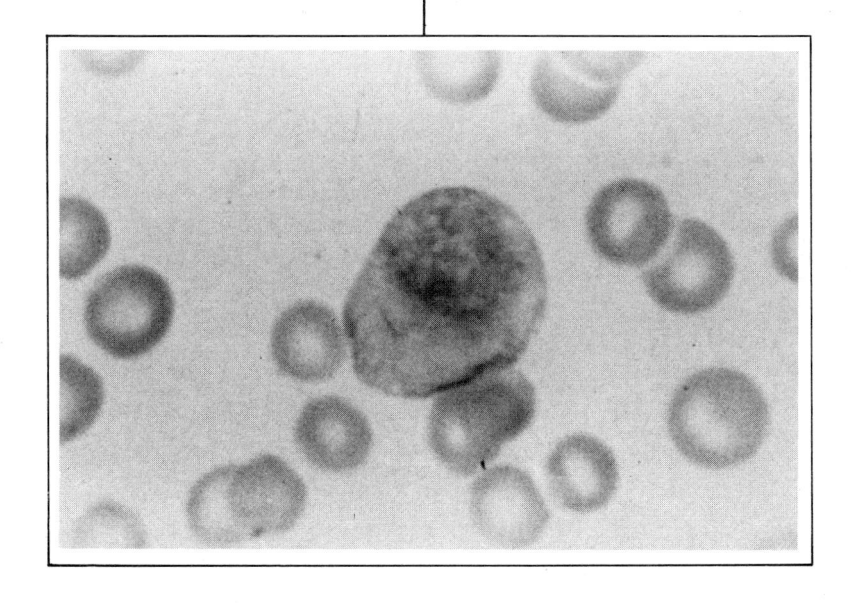

126. The neutrophil shown below is most likely to be found in association with

(A) folic acid deficiency
(B) infection
(C) iron deficiency
(D) malignancy
(E) ingestion of a marrow-toxic agent

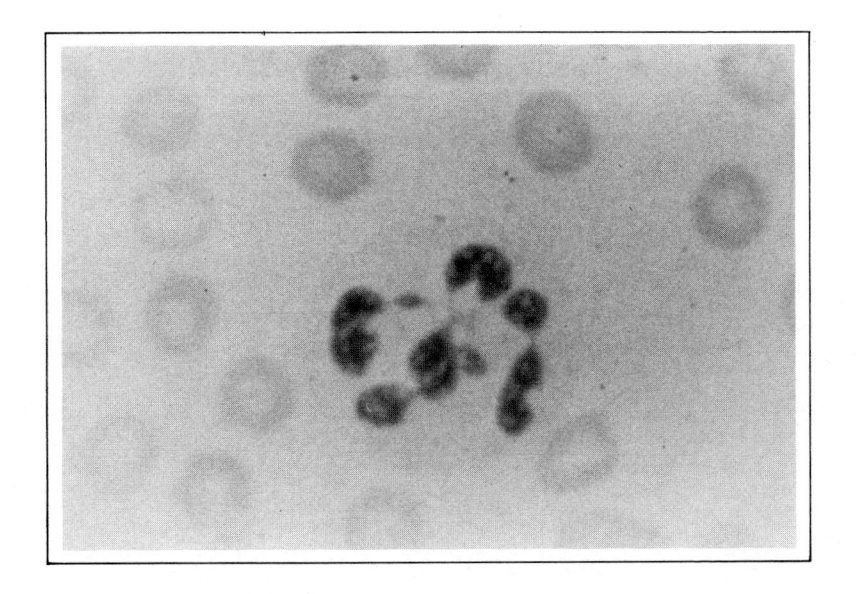

127. The nucleated cell, shown on the facing page located next to the neutrophil, has a gray-pink cytoplasm and is

(A) a polychromatophilic megaloblast
(B) a plasma cell
(C) an orthochromophilic normoblast
(D) a myelocyte
(E) a myeloblast

128. The white blood cells shown on the facing page are

(A) myeloblasts
(B) monoblasts
(C) lymphoblasts
(D) atypical lymphocytes
(E) plasmablasts

Photograph accompanies Question 127

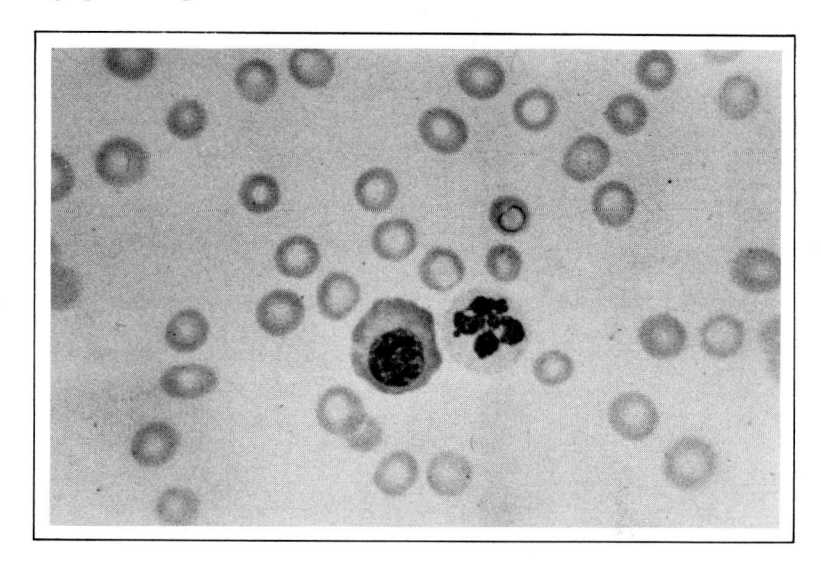

Photograph accompanies Question 128

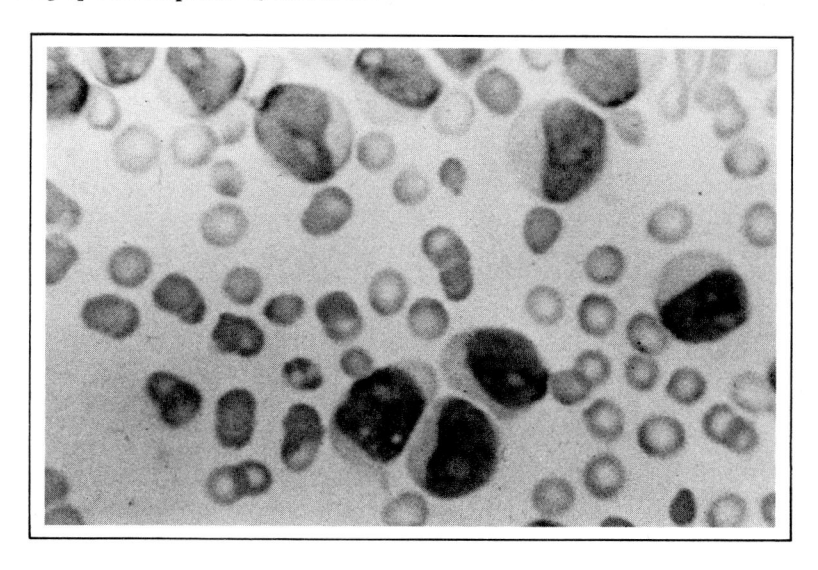

129. The photomicrograph below shows a specimen of joint fluid observed through a polarizing microscope. The crystals observed exhibit positive birefringence. Based on their appearance and polarizing properties, the crystals are composed of

(A) talcum powder
(B) monosodium urate
(C) cholesterol
(D) calcium oxalate monohydrate
(E) calcium pyrophosphate dihydrate

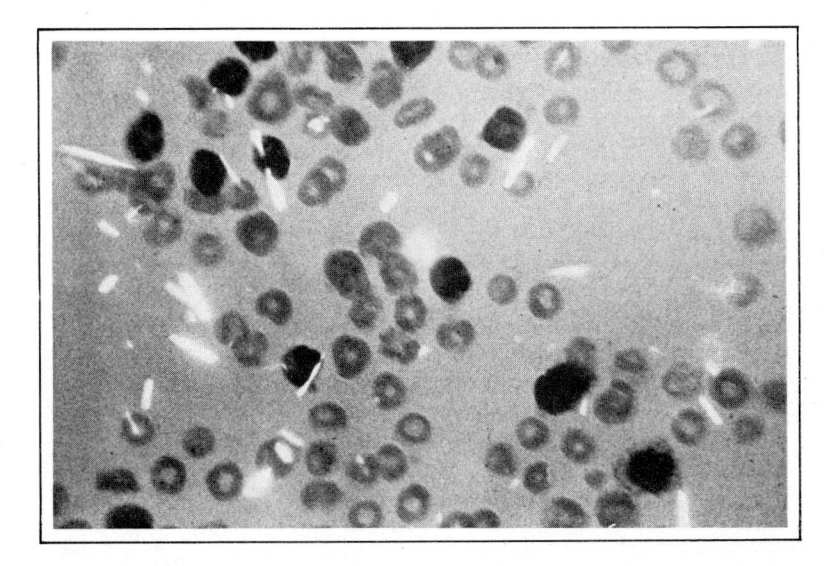

130. The cluster of cells shown on the facing page is from the bone marrow of a patient with

(A) Hodgkin's disease
(B) erythroleukemia
(C) Waldenström's macroglobulinemia
(D) multiple myeloma
(E) metastatic carcinoma

131. The photograph on the facing page shows an unstained drop of blood mixed with two drops of sodium metabisulfite and incubated for thirty minutes. The red cells contain

(A) hemoglobin A
(B) hemoglobin A_2
(C) hemoglobin C
(D) hemoglobin F
(E) hemoglobin S

Photograph accompanies Question 130

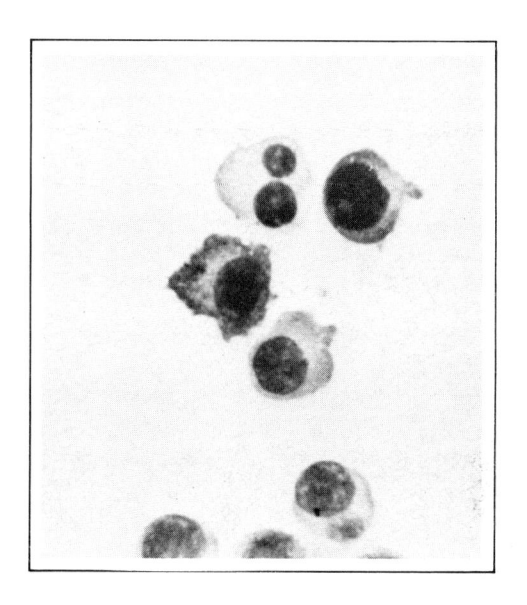

Photograph accompanies Question 131

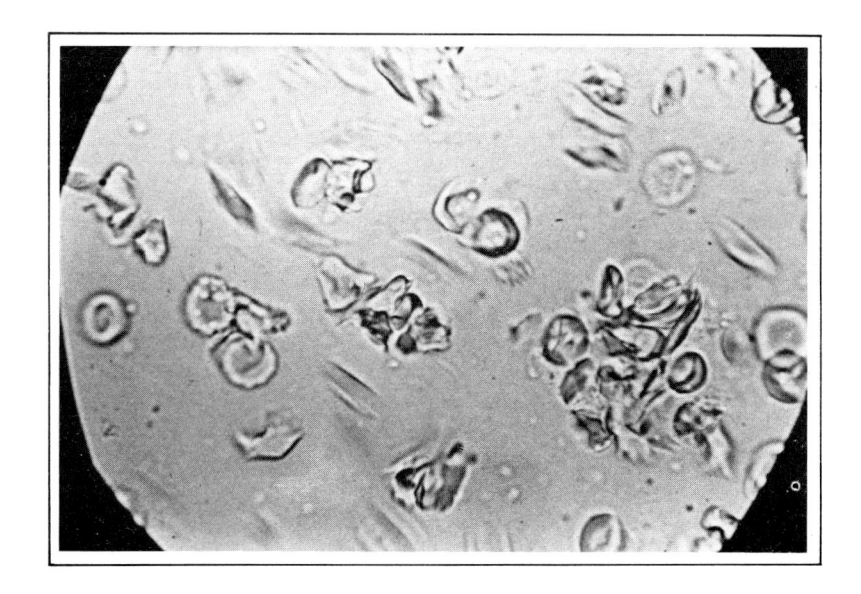

132. The representative region from a bone marrow aspirate, shown below, taken from a 70-year-old man with weakness and anemia is most consistent with a diagnosis of

(A) monomyelocytic leukemia
(B) histiocytic lymphoma
(C) multiple myeloma (plasma cell dyscrasia)
(D) Gaucher's disease
(E) hairy cell leukemia

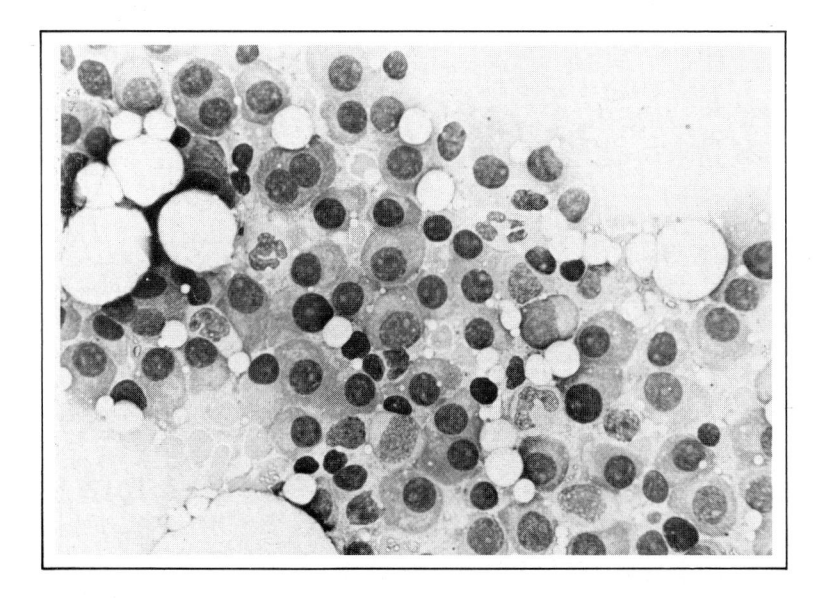

133. Which of the following laboratory findings is LEAST likely to be present in a patient with sickle cell anemia?

(A) Normochromic anemia
(B) Increased number of target cells
(C) Elevated reticulocyte count
(D) Elevated sedimentation rate
(E) Increased hemoglobin F

134. Patients with sickle cell trait have which of the following genotypes?

(A) α^s α β β
(B) α^s α^s β β
(C) α α β β^s
(D) α α β^s β^s
(E) α α^s β β^s

Questions 135-136

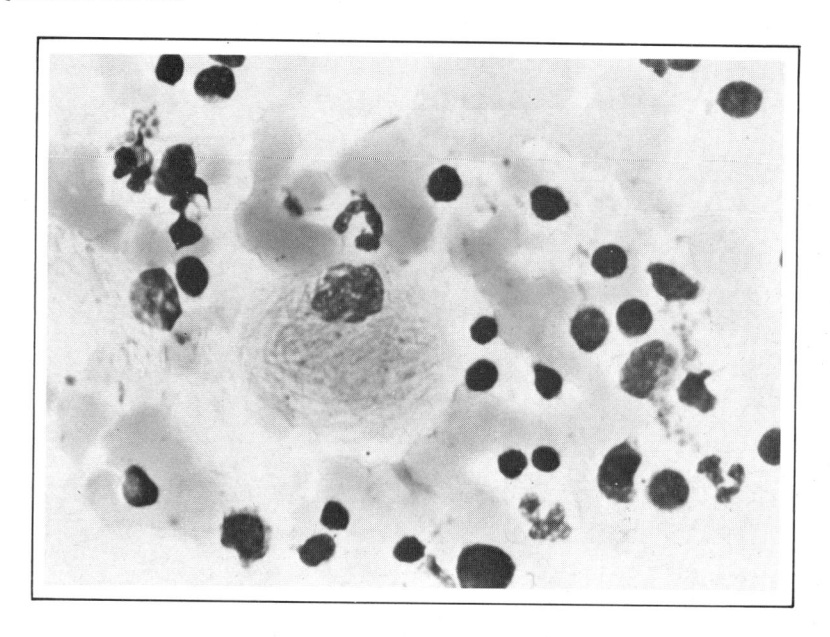

135. The cell shown above was found in a bone marrow aspiration from a 25-year-old man. It is most compatible with a diagnosis of

(A) Niemann-Pick disease
(B) histiocytic lymphoma
(C) megaloblastic anemia
(D) Gaucher's disease
(E) myelogenous leukemia

136. All of the following statements concerning the disease associated with the cell shown above are true EXCEPT

(A) the cells are typically 20 to 100 microns in diameter and have a wrinkled, striated cytoplasm
(B) inheritance is autosomal dominant with variable penetrance
(C) serum acid phosphatase is frequently elevated
(D) an excess amount of sphingolipid is stored in body tissues
(E) the disease rarely involves the nervous system resulting in early death

Questions 137-138

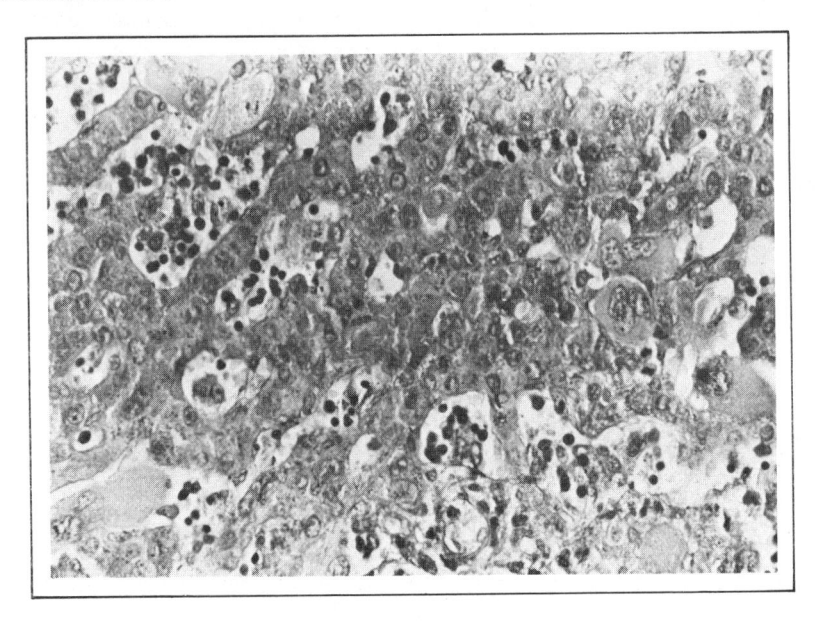

137. The pathologic process depicted in the high-power photomicrograph of a section of liver shown above is compatible with a diagnosis of

(A) acute viral hepatitis
(B) hepatic cirrhosis
(C) extramedullary hematopoiesis
(D) alcoholic hepatitis
(E) common bile duct obstruction

138. The extrahepatic systemic disease most likely to produce the sinusoidal infiltrate shown above is

(A) acute myelomonocytic leukemia
(B) porphyria
(C) hemosiderosis
(D) rheumatoid arthritis
(E) myelofibrosis with myeloid metaplasia

139. Which of the following causes of megaloblastic anemia is NOT usually associated with vitamin B_{12} deficiency?

(A) Blind loop syndrome
(B) *Diphyllobothrium latum* infestation
(C) Alcoholic liver disease
(D) Gastric atrophy
(E) Total gastrectomy

140. Vitamin K is a necessary co-factor for the synthesis of all of the following EXCEPT

(A) prothrombin
(B) clotting factor V
(C) clotting factor VIII
(D) clotting factor IX
(E) clotting factor X

141. Which of the following substances inhibits platelet aggregation?

(A) Prostaglandin E
(B) Epinephrine
(C) Adenosine diphosphate
(D) 5-Hydroxytryptamine
(E) Thrombin

142. The normal red blood cell survival time in humans is approximately

(A) 30 days
(B) 60 days
(C) 90 days
(D) 120 days
(E) 150 days

143. Excessive red blood cell lysis by complement in the presence of acidified serum should suggest a diagnosis of

(A) hemolytic uremic syndrome
(B) acute intermittent porphyria
(C) paroxysmal nocturnal hemoglobinuria
(D) pyruvate kinase deficiency
(E) Goodpasture's syndrome

144. Typical findings in a patient with von Willebrand's disease, include all of the following EXCEPT

(A) decreased levels of factor VIII
(B) decreased glass bead adhesion of platelets
(C) prolonged bleeding time
(D) frequent hemarthrosis and spontaneous joint hemorrhage
(E) menorrhagia

145. The osmotic fragility pattern depicted by the dotted line in the figure below is most suggestive of

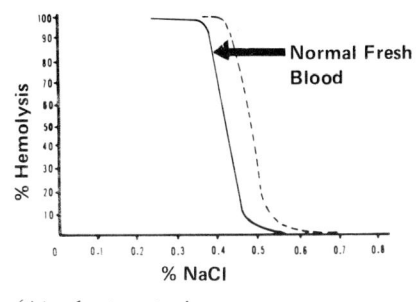

(A) leptocytosis
(B) β-thalassemia
(C) iron deficiency anemia
(D) sickle cell anemia
(E) hereditary spherocytosis

146. Delta-aminolevulinic acid is excreted in increased amounts in the urine of patients with

(A) lead poisoning
(B) carcinoma of the pancreas
(C) chronic pyelonephritis
(D) vitamin C intoxication
(E) ulcerative colitis

147. Heparin acts to inhibit coagulation by all of the following mechanisms EXCEPT

(A) inhibiting vitamin K dependent enzymes
(B) inhibiting thrombin
(C) inhibiting platelet function
(D) inhibiting factor Xa
(E) increasing fibrinolysis

148. A chromosomal abnormality is associated with which of the following neoplastic processes?

(A) Acute lymphoblastic leukemia
(B) Acute myelogenous leukemia
(C) Chronic myelogenous leukemia
(D) Polycythemia vera
(E) Multiple myeloma

149. Lymphocytic predominant Hodgkin's disease was diagnosed in biopsies of the left axillary and mediastinal lymph nodes of a young man who presented with fever, weight loss, and night sweats. He had no other sites of Hodgkin's disease infiltration. His disease would be classed as stage

(A) I A
(B) I B
(C) II B
(D) III B
(E) IV B

150. Sézary cells may be found in the peripheral blood of patients with which of the following diseases?

(A) Acute lymphoblastic leukemia
(B) Burkitt's lymphoma
(C) Multiple myeloma
(D) Acute monocytic leukemia
(E) Mycosis fungoides

151. A patient with Waldenström's macroglobulinemia would commonly have all of the following findings EXCEPT

(A) elevated serum viscosity
(B) sheet-like infiltrates of plasma cells in bone marrow
(C) rouleau formation on peripheral smear
(D) anemia
(E) monoclonal gammopathy

152. The leukocyte alkaline phosphatase (LAP) level is particularly low in which of the following conditions?

(A) Myocardial infarction
(B) Acute lymphoblastic leukemia
(C) Leukemoid reaction
(D) Chronic granulocytic leukemia
(E) Idiopathic thrombocythemia

153. Approximately what percentage of transferrin is saturated with iron in the serum of a normal individual?

(A) 10 percent
(B) 33 percent
(C) 50 percent
(D) 66 percent
(E) 90 percent

154. An anemic patient has the following red cell indices: mean corpuscular volume, 70 cu μm; mean corpuscular hemoglobin, 22 g/100 ml; mean corpuscular hemoglobin concentration, 34%. The values are most consistent with a diagnosis of

(A) folic acid deficiency anemia
(B) iron deficiency anemia
(C) pernicious anemia
(D) thalassemia minor
(E) sideroblastic anemia

155. Chronic myelogenous leukemia is LEAST likely to be associated with

(A) thrombocytopenia
(B) basophilia
(C) splenomegaly
(D) mild anemia (hemoglobin, 12 g/100 ml)
(E) leukocyte count greater than 50,000/cu mm

156. Antimalarial therapy with primaquine may cause an acute hemolytic episode in individuals with

(A) iron deficiency anemia
(B) sickle cell anemia
(C) hereditary elliptocytosis
(D) pyruvate kinase deficiency
(E) glucose 6-phosphate dehydrogenase deficiency

157. Neutropenia associated with leukocyte autoantibody is characteristic of

(A) carcinoma of the colon
(B) uremic pericarditis
(C) Felty's syndrome
(D) severe burns
(E) myocardial infarction

158. A young child has recurrent bacterial infections, eczema, thrombocytopenia, lymphadenopathy, and the absence of delayed-type hypersensitivity. The most likely diagnosis is

(A) Pelger-Hüet anomaly
(B) Wiskott-Aldrich syndrome
(C) Chédiak-Higashi syndrome
(D) chronic granulomatous disease of childhood
(E) nodular-sclerosing Hodgkin's disease

159. Which of the following conditions is most likely to cause rupture of the spleen?

(A) Hodgkin's disease
(B) Malaria
(C) Trauma
(D) Thrombocytopenia
(E) Acanthosis

DIRECTIONS: Each question below contains four suggested answers of which **one** or **more** is correct. Choose the answer

A	if	**1, 2, and 3**	are correct
B	if	**1 and 3**	are correct
C	if	**2 and 4**	are correct
D	if	**4**	is correct
E	if	**1, 2, 3, and 4**	are correct

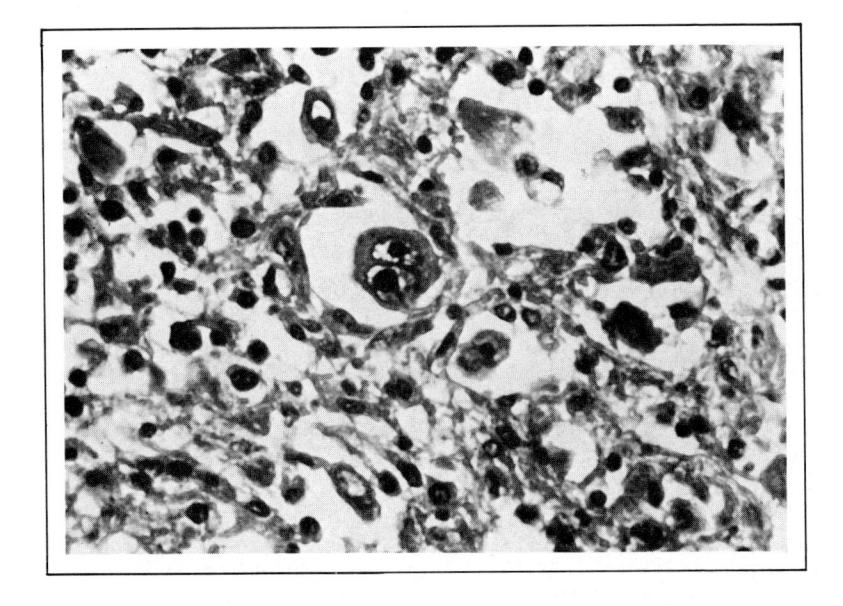

160. The binucleated or bilobed tumor giant cell with prominent acidophilic "owl-eye" nucleoli shown above

(1) is necessary, but not sufficient for the diagnosis of Hodgkin's disease
(2) is sometimes referred to as the "lacunar cell"
(3) may be seen in benign conditions
(4) is a rapidly proliferating tumor cell seen in mid-division

161. Which of the following mechanisms contribute to the decreased erythrocyte survival in autoimmune hemolytic anemia?

(1) Complement mediated lysis
(2) Decreased hemoglobin synthesis
(3) Increased phagocytosis of erythrocytes by the reticuloendothelial system
(4) Hemosiderin deposition

Questions 162-164

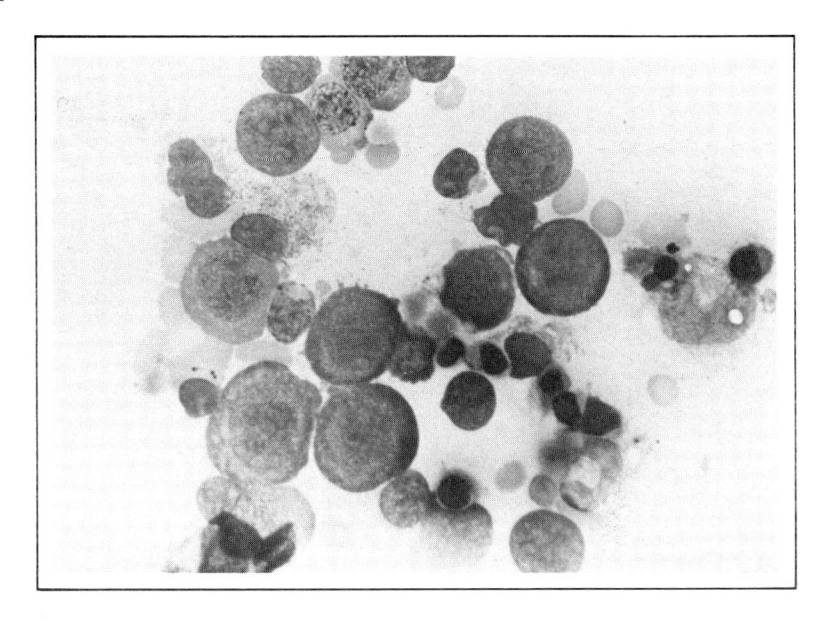

162. Morphologic features in peripheral blood that would be consistent with the megaloblastic bone marrow shown above include

(1) macrocytes with mean corpuscular volumes exceeding 110 cu μm (fl)
(2) numerous myeloblasts
(3) neutrophils with more than the usual three to four segments
(4) secondary polycythemia

163. The megaloblastic red cell colony shown above could be found in bone marrow aspirates from patients who had

(1) erythroleukemia
(2) severe folate and B_{12} deficiency
(3) been treated with anti-folates for leukemia
(4) vitamin A responsive anemia

164. In addition to megaloblastic erythroid changes, findings in the bone marrow aspirate shown above include

(1) decreased myeloid to erythroid ratio (1:1)
(2) giant band forms with maturation arrested in the granulocytic series
(3) increased mitotic figures in red cell precursors
(4) megaloblastic platelet precursors

35

Questions 165-167

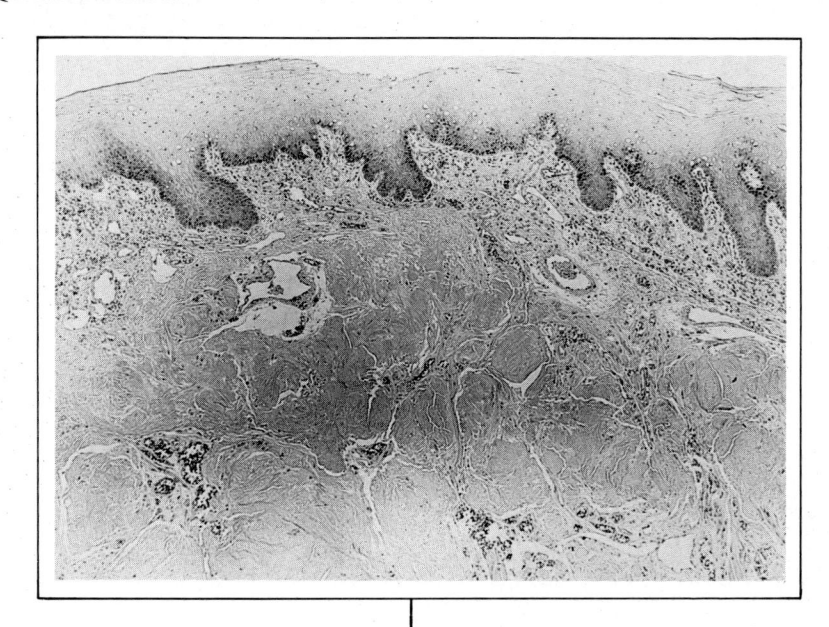

165. The amorphous material deposited in the section of tongue shown above stains pink with Congo red stain and in polarized light appears apple-green in color. Its presence in an elderly man with macroglossia and atypical marrow plasmacytosis would be

(1) unremarkable and occur frequently in the geriatric population
(2) associated with the presence of M-type serum proteins or Bence Jones proteinuria
(3) is almost invariable associated with an increased concentration of normal immunoglobulins
(4) is associated with depositions of similar amorphous material in the heart, ligaments, skin, and peripheral nerves

166. Dependable laboratory studies that would aid in the diagnosis of this process include

(1) serum electrophoresis
(2) rectal biopsy or biopsy of clinically abnormal joint synovium
(3) increased absorption of Congo red and Evans blue dyes from the circulation
(4) immunoelectrophoresis on concentrated urine samples

167. Clinical features associated with primary distribution of this material include

(1) diarrhea and malabsorption
(2) cardiac failure unresponsive to digitalis administration
(3) polyarthritis with thickening of periarticular tissues
(4) peripheral neuropathy

SUMMARY OF DIRECTIONS				
A	B	C	D	E
1, 2, 3 only	1, 3 only	2, 4 only	4 only	All are correct

168. Patients with paroxysmal nocturnal hemoglobinuria may develop

(1) iron deficiency anemia
(2) acute leukemia
(3) venous thrombosis
(4) nephrotic syndrome

169. Enlargement of the spleen is frequently seen in

(1) Gaucher's disease
(2) cirrhosis
(3) infectious mononucleosis
(4) chronic myelogenous leukemia

DIRECTIONS: The group of question in this section consist of five lettered headings followed by several numbered items. For each numbered item choose the **one** lettered heading with which it is **most** closely associated. Each lettered heading may be used once, more than once, or not at all.

Questions 170-174
For each description below, choose the type of leukemia with which it is most likely to be associated

- (A) Acute lymphoblastic leukemia
- (B) Acute myelogenous (granulocytic) leukemia
- (C) Acute promyelocytic leukemia
- (D) Chronic lymphocytic leukemia
- (E) Chronic myelogenous leukemia

170. Auer rods occasionally present in the cytoplasm of leukemic cells

171. Associated with low leukocyte alkaline phosphatase levels and the Philadelphia chromosome

172. High peripheral white cell counts with numerous promyelocytes, myelocytes, metamyelocytes, band forms, polymorphonuclear leukocytes, and eosinophilic and basophilic prescursors

173. Characteristically associated with a short course and diffuse intravascular coagulation

174. Occurs in older adults, produces the fewest symptoms of the group listed and is associated with the longest survival

Cardiovascular System

DIRECTIONS: Each question below contains five suggested answers. Choose the **one best** response to each question.

175. The process illustrated below probably represents

(A) atherosclerotic coronary artery disease with thrombosis
(B) acute polyarteritis nodosa
(C) necrotizing angiitis
(D) syphilitic arteritis
(E) medial calcinosis

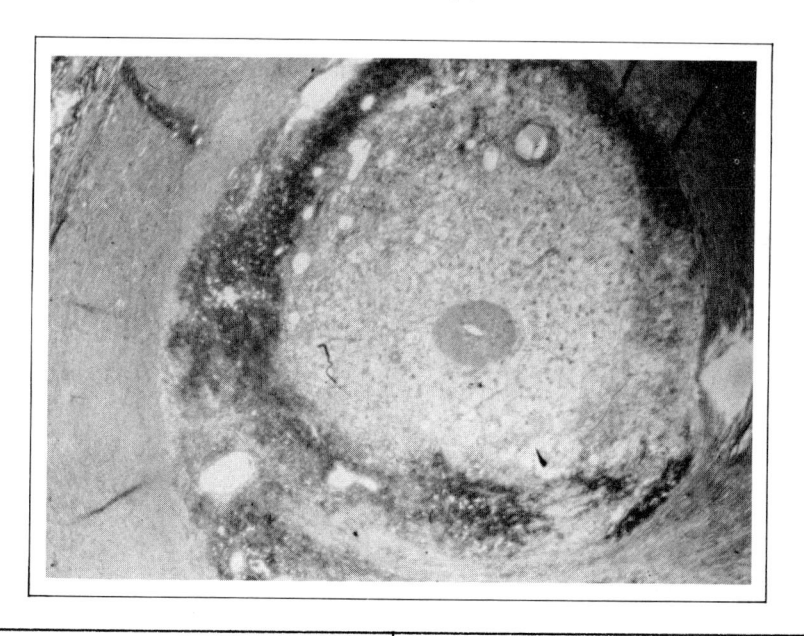

176. Raynaud's disease involves primarily the

(A) myocardium
(B) lung parenchyma
(C) tendons of the hand
(D) cells of the adrenal medulla
(E) small arteries of the extremities

177. Which of the following conditions is most likely to predispose to embolism?

(A) Atrial fibrillation
(B) Pulmonary stenosis
(C) Ventricular septal defect
(D) Aortic stenosis
(E) Atrial septal defect

178. The preponderance of pulmonary emboli arise from the

(A) pelvic veins
(B) veins of the hepatoportal system
(C) veins of the lower leg
(D) veins of the arm
(E) lung from in situ thrombi

179. Acute cor pulmonale is frequently precipitated by

(A) phenylephrine injection
(B) histamine shock
(C) interstitial emphysema
(D) massive pulmonary emboli
(E) bronchiectasis

180. Syphilitic aneurysms of the aorta most commonly are found in the

(A) abdominal part just above the bifurcation
(B) abdominal part directly below the diaphragm
(C) thorax just above the diaphragm
(D) ascending portion of the arch
(E) descending portion of the arch

181. The process illustrated below is usually secondary to

(A) coronary artery atherosclerosis
(B) viral septicemia
(C) cerebral infarction
(D) mural thrombosis
(E) cobalt intoxication

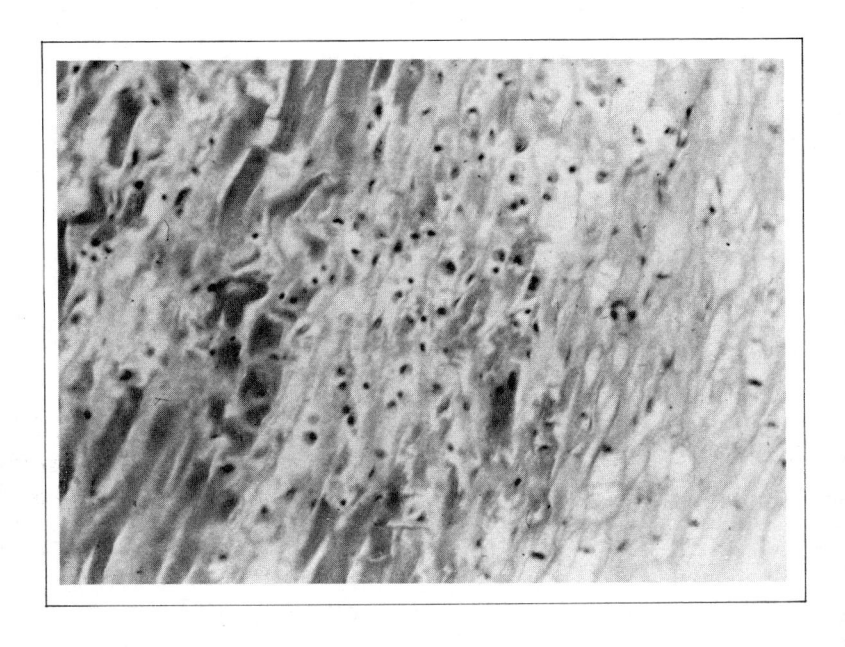

182. The myocardial infarct shown in the pathologic specimen below occurred approximately

(A) 12 hours ago
(B) 72 hours ago
(C) 7 days ago
(D) 14 days ago
(E) 28 days ago

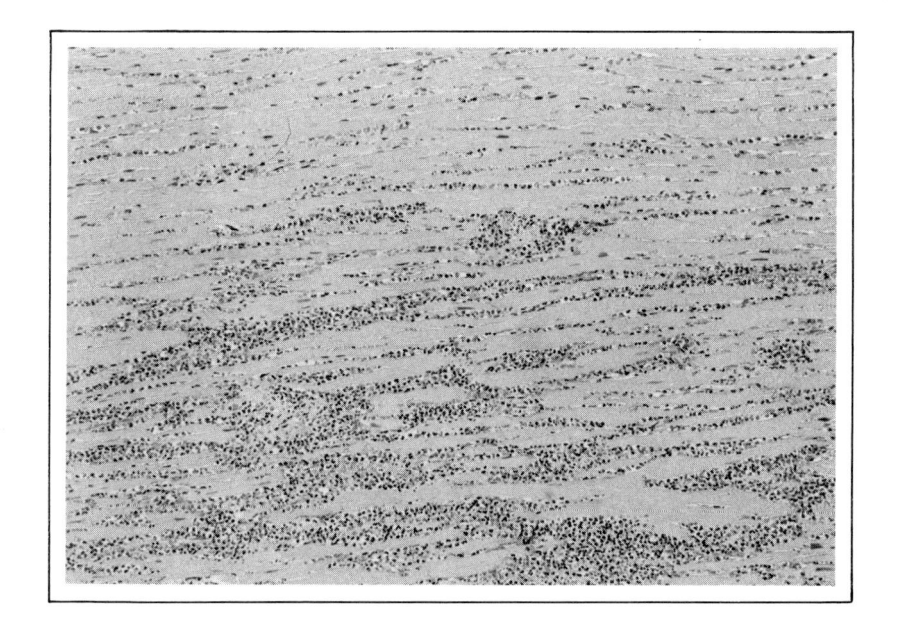

183. The mortality from myocardial infarction is most closely related to the occurrence of

(A) a pericardial effusion
(B) pulmonary edema
(C) coronary artery thrombosis
(D) an arrhythmia
(E) systemic hypotension

184. All patients who die of cardiac arrhythmias complicating myocardial infarction

(A) have a previous history of chest pain radiating down the left arm
(B) do not necessarily have autopsy evidence of coronary artery thrombosis
(C) have a pericardial effusion at autopsy
(D) have at least one macroscopically visible thrombus in a coronary artery
(E) are forewarned by peripheral edema

185. The cardiac lesion present in the ventricular wall of the heart shown below is associated with

(A) acute rheumatic carditis
(B) subacute bacterial endocarditis
(C) acute myocardial infarct
(D) vitamin B_1 (thiamine) deficiency
(E) viral myocarditis

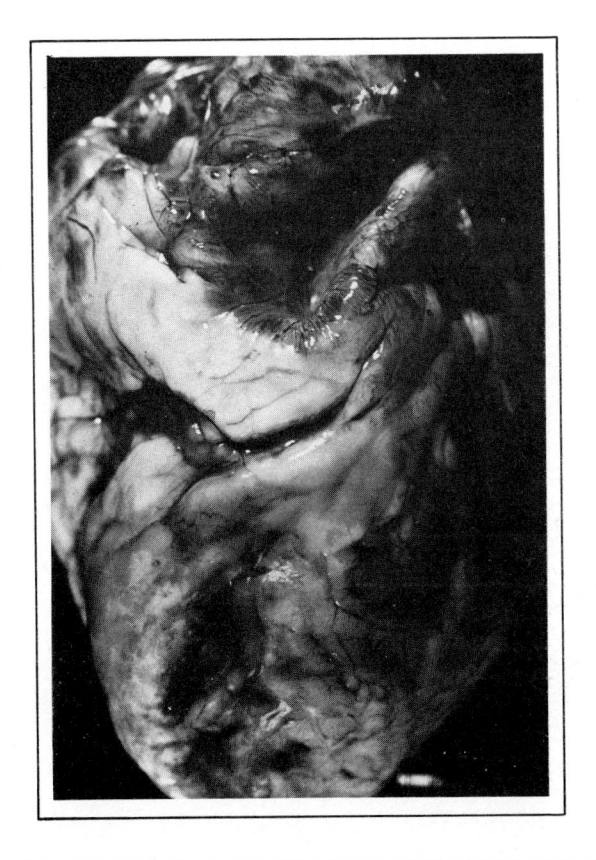

186. Which of the following conditions is not a major manifestation of acute rheumatic fever?

(A) Carditis
(B) Hepatosplenomegaly
(C) Polyarthritis
(D) Chorea
(E) Erythema marginatum

187. The most commonly affected valve in rheumatic fever is

(A) the mitral valve
(B) the aortic valve
(C) the tricuspid valve
(D) the pulmonary valve
(E) either the tricuspid or mitral valve

188. Carditis in acute rheumatic fever typically affects the

(A) endocardium, myocardium, and pericardium
(B) endocardium only
(C) valves only
(D) pericardium only
(E) myocardium only

189. The most common heart defect associated with congenital rubella is

(A) atrial septal defect
(B) patent ductus arteriosus
(C) ventricular septal defect
(D) pulmonary stenosis
(E) tetralogy of Fallot

190. Symptomatic pulmonary valve stenosis is most frequently

(A) congenital
(B) a result of atherosclerotic cardiac disease
(C) a result of rheumatic endocarditis
(D) found in people over 60 years of age
(E) found in women between the ages of 30 and 50

191. Which of the following congenital cardiac lesions, is most frequently involved in bacterial endocarditis?

(A) Atrial septal defect
(B) Ventricular septal defect
(C) Pulmonic stenosis
(D) Tetralogy of Fallot
(E) Patent ductus arteriosus

192. Complete obliteration of the aortic lumen by a coarctation proximal to the ductus arteriosus will be fatal unless

(A) the foramen ovale is closed
(B) the ductus is ligated
(C) pulmonary stenosis coexists
(D) the ductus remains patent
(E) the tricuspid valve is incompetent

193. The necrotizing arteritis of the small muscular artery shown below is most likely to be due to

(A) myasthenia gravis
(B) polyarteritis nodosa
(C) atherosclerosis
(D) dissecting aneurysm
(E) syphilis

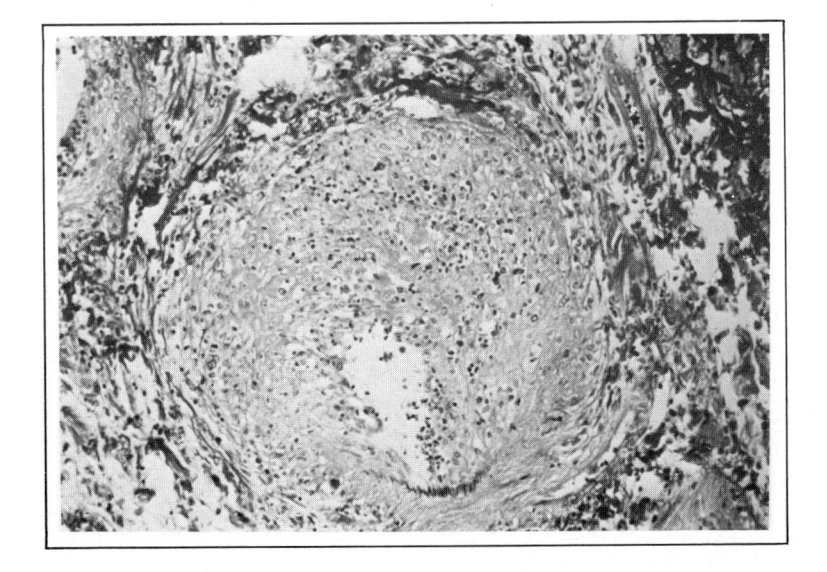

DIRECTIONS: Each question below contains four suggested answers of which **one** or **more** is correct. Choose the answer

A	if	1, 2, and 3	are correct
B	if	1 and 3	are correct
C	if	2 and 4	are correct
D	if	4	is correct
E	if	1, 2, 3, and 4	are correct

194. Mönckeberg's medial calcific sclerosis

(1) affects muscular arteries
(2) affects veins
(3) is common after the age of 50
(4) is common in the descending aorta

195. Which of the following conditions are thought to play a role in dissecting aortic aneurysm?

(1) Arteriosclerosis
(2) Hypertension
(3) Syphilitic aortitis
(4) Cystic medial necrosis

196. A patient with Raynaud's disease, only, will present with

(1) calcinosis
(2) telangiectasia
(3) sclerodactyly
(4) cold sensitivity of the fingers

197. Types of pericarditis that can often lead to a fibrosing, constrictive pericarditis include

(1) staphylococcal
(2) rheumatic
(3) mycobacterial
(4) uremic

198. Myocardial infarction occurs most frequently in the

(1) interventricular septum
(2) right anterolateral wall
(3) left ventricle
(4) posterior right ventricle

199. Valvular verrucae found in rheumatic carditis patients

(1) are precipitates of fibrin and platelets
(2) occur along the free margin of the valve
(3) usually do not contain bacteria
(4) characteristically reveal Aschoff bodies on histologic examination

200. Congenital cardiac lesions that are associated with cyanosis include

(1) tetralogy of Fallot
(2) patent ductus arteriosus
(3) transposition of the great vessels
(4) atrial septal defect

SUMMARY OF DIRECTIONS

A	B	C	D	E
1, 2, 3 only	1, 3 only	2, 4 only	4 only	All are correct

201. Severe mitral stenosis, as shown below, is frequently accompanied by

(1) severe left ventricular hypertrophy
(2) left atrial enlargement with atrial fibrillation
(3) pulmonary stenosis (valvular)
(4) chronic passive pulmonary congestion

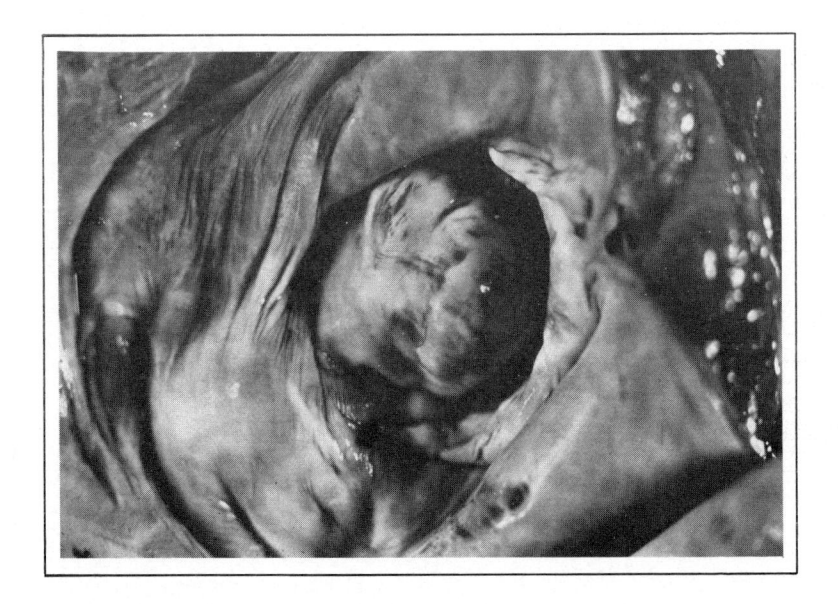

202. The tetralogy of Fallot includes which of the following cardiac anomalies?

(1) Pulmonic stenosis
(2) Right ventricular hypertrophy
(3) Dextroposition of the aorta
(4) Tricuspid insufficiency

203. Signs of pericardial inflammation may be seen in

(1) acute myocardial infarction
(2) rheumatic fever
(3) uremia
(4) aortic stenosis

46

DIRECTIONS: The groups of questions in this section consist of five lettered headings followed by several numbered items. For each numbered item choose the **one** lettered heading with which it is **most** closely associated. Each lettered heading may be used once, more than once, or not at all.

Questions 204-207
For each cardiac condition, choose the infectious agent with which it is most likely to be associated.

(A) Coxsackievirus
(B) *Mycobacterium tuberculosis*
(C) *Streptococcus*
(D) *Treponema*
(E) *Escherichia coli*

204. Primary myocarditis

205. Rheumatic fever

206. Aortic aneurysms

207. Suppurative pericarditis

Questions 208-211
For each of the following descriptions, choose the type of myocarditis with which it is most likely to be associated.

(A) Chagas' disease associated myocarditis
(B) Rheumatic (interstitial) myocarditis
(C) Acute, idiopathic myocarditis of Fiedler
(D) Viral myocarditis
(E) Acute suppurative myocarditis

208. Aschoff bodies

209. Predominantly chronic myocarditis endemic in portions of South America

210. Myocardial lesions include giant cells, granulomatous infiltrates, eosinophils, lymphocytic cells, and plasma cells

211. Frequent in newborn or young infants

Questions 212-214
For each aneurysm, choose its usual anatomic location.

(A) Thoracic aorta
(B) Abdominal aorta
(C) Renal arteries
(D) Temporal arteries
(E) Cerebral arteries

212. Berry aneurysm

213. Arteriosclerotic aneurysm

214. Syphilitic aneurysm

Question 215-217
For each histologic feature, choose the arterial lesion with which it is most likely to be associated.

(A) Granulomatous inflammation in the region of the internal elastic membrane
(B) Intimal lipid accumulation
(C) Necrotizing inflammation of the muscular media
(D) Ring-like calcification within the media of muscular arteries
(E) Polymorphonuclear leukocyte infiltration of all vessel layers with mural thrombosis

215. Atherosclerosis

216. Giant cell arteritis

217. Polyarteritis nodosa

Respiratory System

218. A patient presents with hemoptysis and acute renal failure. A diagnosis consistent with this clinical picture is

(A) asbestosis
(B) primary atypical pneumonia
(C) Goodpasture's syndrome
(D) tuberculosis
(E) Weil's disease

219. Alpha$_1$-antitrypsin deficiency is associated with

(A) thalassemia
(B) nephrotic syndrome
(C) panlobular emphysema
(D) anthracosis
(E) renal cell carcinoma

220. Enlargement of pulmonary alveolar spaces with destruction of septal walls is the definition of

(A) chronic bronchitis
(B) emphysema
(C) pulmonary infarction
(D) pulmonary hypertension
(E) alveolar proteinosis

221. A chest x-ray that shows a shaggy cavity with a thick irregular border and satellite densities in the right lower lobe is most compatible with

(A) histoplasmosis
(B) bronchogenic carcinoma
(C) tuberculosis
(D) *Nocardia asteroides*
(E) abscess

222. The pathogenesis of extrinsic asthma is most similar to that of

(A) emphysema
(B) bronchopneumonia
(C) Goodpasture's syndrome
(D) hay fever
(E) oat cell carcinoma

223. An illness initially characterized by cough, tightness in the chest, and breathlessness occurring on return to work but improving during working days is probably

(A) byssinosis
(B) bagassosis
(C) silicosis
(D) coal worker's pneumoconiosis
(E) asbestosis

224. The presence of numerous metaplastic squamous cells in the cytology sample shown below, obtained from the lower respiratory tract, suggests

(A) squamous cell carcinoma
(B) oat cell carcinoma
(C) reaction to chronic irritation
(D) acute bronchopneumonia
(E) a normal respiratory tract

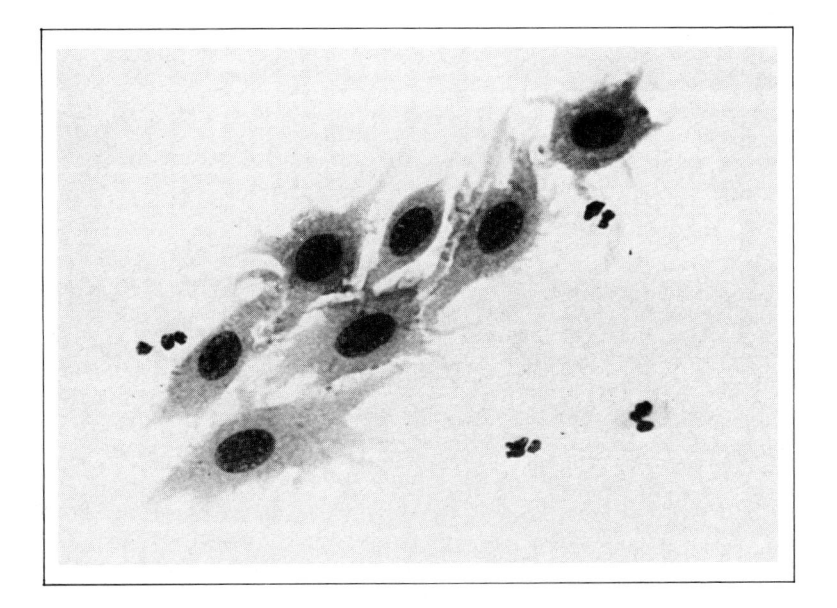

225. The organism that is most likely to cause the necrotizing pulmonary lesion shown on the facing page is

(A) *Pseudomonas aeruginosa*
(B) *Mycobacterium tuberculosis*
(C) *Pneumocystis carinii*
(D) *Trichinella spiralis*
(E) *Candida albicans*

226. The lung biopsy, shown on the facing page, stained with methenamine silver (Grocott) was removed from a 10-year-old child with acute lymphoblastic leukemia, who developed a patchy pulmonary infiltrate and respiratory insufficiency. The most likely diagnosis is

(A) *Pseudomonas* pneumonia
(B) *Aspergillus* pneumonia
(C) *Pneumocystis carinii* pneumonia
(D) pneumococcal pneumonia
(E) influenza pneumonia

Photograph accompanies Question 225

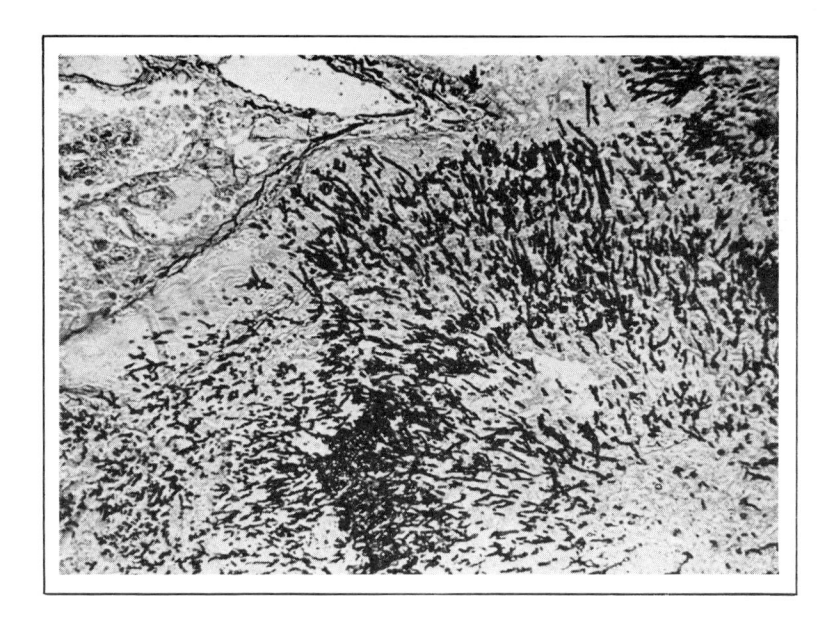

Photograph accompanies Question 226

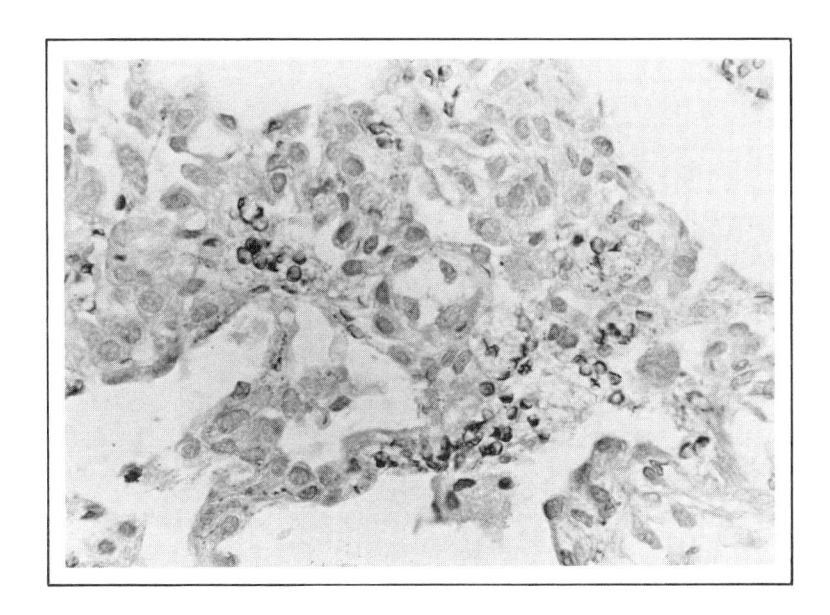

227. The histologic type of bronchogenic carcinoma most commonly associated with nonmetastatic endocrine manifestations is

(A) adenocarcinoma
(B) oat cell carcinoma
(C) large cell carcinoma
(D) anaplastic carcinoma
(E) epidermoid carcinoma

228. Which primary, malignant, pulmonary tumor most frequently arises in a scar?

(A) Epidermoid carcinoma
(B) Adenoid cystic carcinoma
(C) Small cell undifferentiated (oat cell) carcinoma
(D) Mesothelioma
(E) Adenocarcinoma

DIRECTIONS: Each question below contains four suggested answers of which **one** or **more** is correct. Choose the answer

A	if	1, 2, and 3	are	correct
B	if	1 and 3	are	correct
C	if	2 and 4	are	correct
D	if	4	is	correct
E	if	1, 2, 3, and 4	are	correct

---

229. Cigarette smoking has been linked directly to which of the following pathologic conditions of the bronchi?

(1) Squamous metaplasia
(2) Bronchiectasis
(3) Destruction of normal ciliary action
(4) Bronchopneumonia

230. Conditions that predispose to the development of bronchiectasis include

(1) asthma
(2) chronic sinusitis
(3) avitaminosis A
(4) fibrocystic disease

231. Caseous necrosis is found in

(1) lupus erythematosus
(2) pneumonia
(3) carcinoma
(4) tuberculosis

232. In sarcoidosis, the enlarged hilar lymph nodes

(1) are bilateral
(2) almost never calcify
(3) occur early in the course of the disease
(4) generally regress over a period of time

233. Complications of severe, diffuse panacinar emphysema may include

(1) respiratory acidosis
(2) acute and chronic peptic ulcer disease
(3) right-sided heart failure
(4) pneumothorax

234. "Usual interstitial pneumonia" (fibrosing alveolitis) is characterized by

(1) pulmonary insufficiency and death occurring within a year of the onset of symptoms
(2) cellular thickening of alveolar walls with fibrosis and chronic inflammatory infiltrates
(3) an increased incidence of primary pulmonary malignancy
(4) alveolar-capillary block

235. Pulmonary interstitial fibrosis is reported to result from the use of

(1) busulfan
(2) nitrofurantoin
(3) methysergide
(4) oxygen

236. In primary tuberculosis, the Ghon complex consists of *Mycobacterium tuberculosis* infecting which of the following areas?

(1) Bone marrow
(2) Subpleural pulmonary parenchyma
(3) Kidneys
(4) Tracheobronchial lymph nodes

237. Extrapulmonary manifestations of bronchogenic carcinoma include

(1) Cushing's syndrome
(2) inappropriate antidiuretic hormone activity
(3) peripheral neuropathy and myopathy
(4) cortical cerebellar degeneration

Questions 238-239

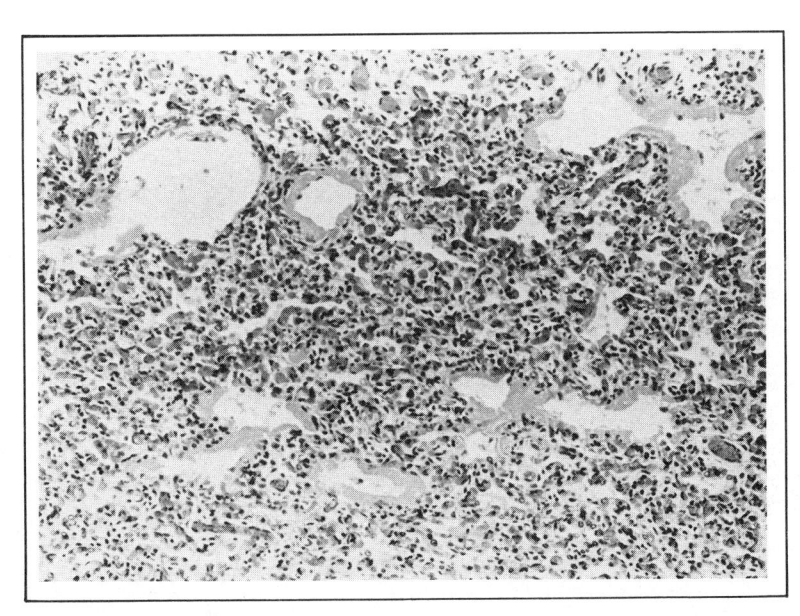

238. The pathologic process shown above was found at autopsy in a four-day-old premature infant. It is consistent with

(1) congenital syphilis
(2) extralobar pulmonary sequestration
(3) primary fungal pneumonitis
(4) respiratory distress syndrome (hyaline membrane disease)

239. A similar pathologic picture can be seen in lungs from adults with

(1) viral pneumonia
(2) uremia
(3) pulmonary irradiation
(4) severe bacterial infection

SUMMARY OF DIRECTIONS				
A	B	C	D	E
1, 2, 3 only	1, 3 only	2, 4 only	4 only	All are correct

240. Pulmonary infarcts

(1) may be due to pulmonary embolism
(2) may be due to septic vasculitis
(3) are hemorrhagic
(4) occur in patients with normal cardiovascular function

DIRECTIONS: The groups of questions in this section consist of five lettered headings followed by several numbered items. For each numbered item choose the **one** lettered heading with which it is **most** closely associated. Each lettered heading may be used once, more than once, or not at all.

Questions 241-244
For each of the pathologic conditions, choose the predominant material that would be found in the affected alveolar spaces.

(A) Edematous fluid
(B) Lipid-laden macrophages
(C) Polymorphonuclear leukocytes
(D) Blood
(E) Hyphae

241. Goodpasture's syndrome

242. Acute left heart failure

243. Lipid pneumonia

244. Acute bronchopneumonia

Questions 245-248
For each tumor, choose its most common site of origin.

(A) Pleura
(B) Bronchial lining
(C) Submucosal bronchial glands
(D) Alveolar lining cells
(E) Bronchial lymphatics

245. Squamous cell carcinoma

246. Alveolar cell carcinoma

247. Adenoid cystic carcinoma

248. Mesothelioma

Gastrointestinal System

DIRECTIONS: Each question below contains five suggested answers. Choose the **one best** response to each question.

249. Which of the following conditions is most likely to be associated with gastric carcinoma?

(A) Pernicious anemia
(B) Alcoholism
(C) Obesity
(D) Hemochromatosis
(E) Duodenal ulcer

250. Transmural inflammation of the intestinal wall with formation of noncaseating granulomas is most typical of

(A) regional enteritis (Crohn's disease)
(B) ulcerative colitis
(C) sarcoidosis
(D) systemic sclerosis
(E) adenocarcinoma

251. Malabsorption is a common feature of all of the following EXCEPT

(A) celiac disease (gluten enteropathy)
(B) tropical sprue
(C) villous adenoma
(D) pancreatic insufficiency
(E) biliary obstruction

252. Peptic duodenal ulcers

(A) occur in patients with achlorhydria
(B) are usually multiple
(C) develop into cancer
(D) are more common in males
(E) never cause hemorrhage

253. The most common tumor of the appendix is

(A) malignant melanoma
(B) adenocarcinoma
(C) argentaffinoma (carcinoid)
(D) lymphoma
(E) fibrosarcoma

254. Chronic passive congestion of the liver with central hemorrhagic necrosis and sclerosis are found in association with

(A) chronic cholecystitis
(B) Dubin-Johnson syndrome
(C) chronic right-sided cardiac failure
(D) cholangitis
(E) leptospirosis (Weil's disease)

255. Adenocarcinoma of the colon, pictured below arising in a villous adenoma, also occurs with increased frequency in association with

(A) polypoid adenoma
(B) hemorrhoids
(C) chronic ulcerative colitis
(D) diverticulosis
(E) Meckel's diverticulum

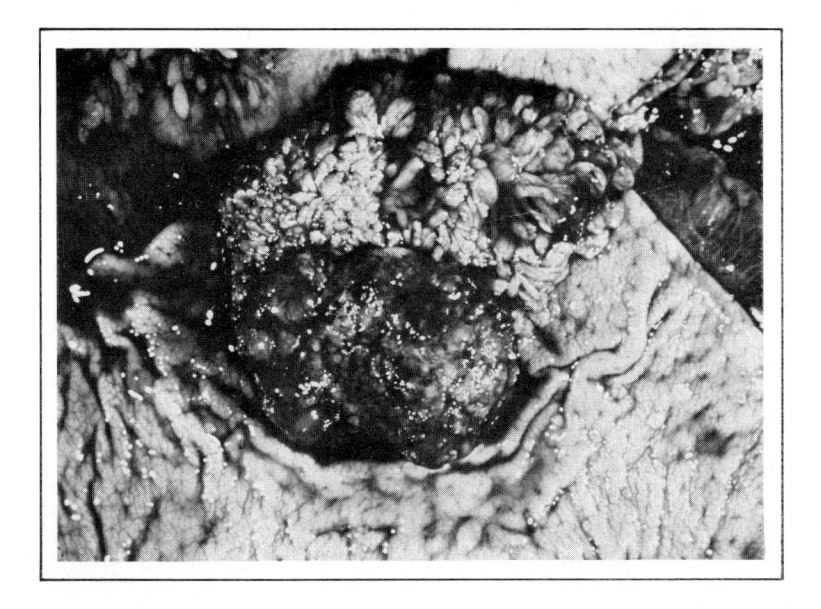

256. Diagnostic criteria for acute alcoholic hepatitis include all of the following EXCEPT

(A) fatty change
(B) alcoholic hyaline
(C) hepatocyte necrosis
(D) portal cirrhosis
(E) acute inflammatory infiltrates

257. The most common tumor found in the liver at autopsy is

(A) hemangioma
(B) hepatocellular carcinoma
(C) metastatic malignancy
(D) cholangiocarcinoma
(E) adenoma

258. The distal colonic biopsy shown below was taken from a 28-year-old Puerto Rican man. The most likely diagnosis is

(A) clonorchiasis
(B) enterobiasis
(C) filariasis
(D) strongyloidiasis
(E) schistosomiasis

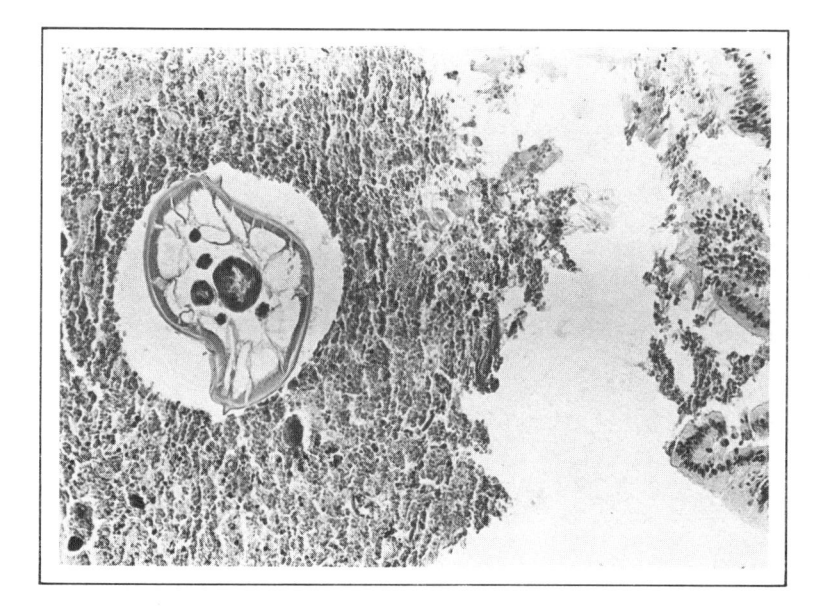

259. Primary carcinoma of the gallbladder is most commonly associated with

(A) carcinoma of the pancreas
(B) carcinoma of the lung
(C) cholelithiasis
(D) hepatitis
(E) Laennec's cirrhosis

260. Most pancreatic carcinomas arise in the

(A) head of the pancreas
(B) body of the pancreas
(C) tail of the pancreas
(D) pancreatic ducts
(E) ectopic pancreatic tissues

261. The ulcerated mucosal lesion at the anorectal junction, shown below, is probably

(A) a villous adenoma
(B) an epidermoid carcinoma
(C) a hemorrhoid
(D) a polypoid adenoma
(E) a mesenteric thrombosis

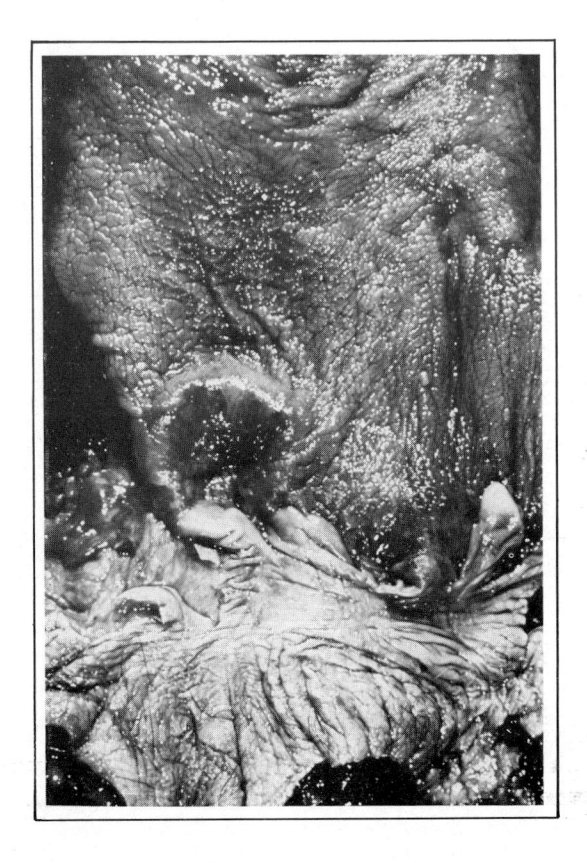

262. A mononuclear portal inflammatory infiltrate which disrupts the limiting plate and surrounds individual hepatocytes (piecemeal necrosis), as shown below, is characteristic of

(A) ascending cholangitis
(B) chronic active hepatitis
(C) acute alcoholic hepatitis
(D) cholestatic jaundice
(E) nutritional cirrhosis

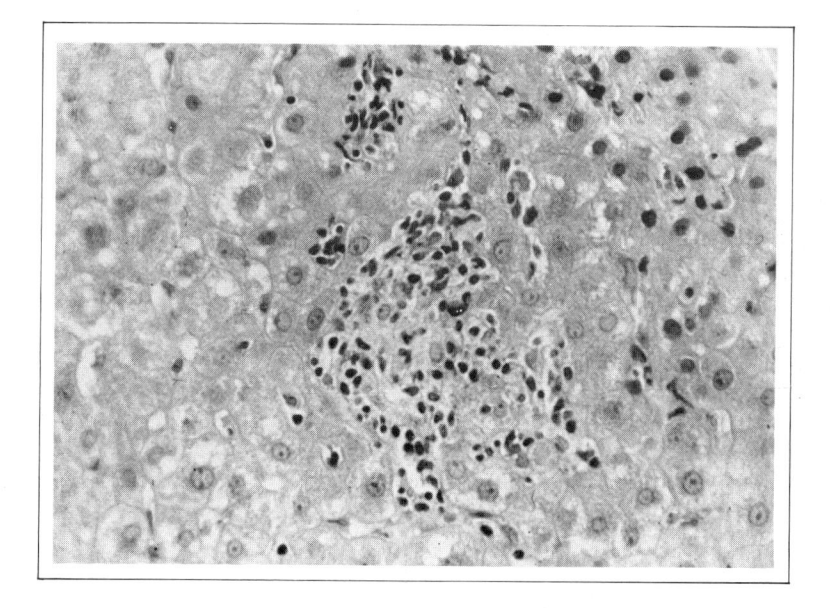

263. Meckel's diverticulum occurs in the

(A) duodenum
(B) esophagus
(C) colon
(D) ileum
(E) jejunum

DIRECTIONS: Each question below contains four suggested answers of which **one** or **more** is correct. Choose the answer

A	if	1, 2, and 3	are correct
B	if	1 and 3	are correct
C	if	2 and 4	are correct
D	if	4	is correct
E	if	1, 2, 3, and 4	are correct

264. Congenital pyloric stenosis

(1) occurs almost always in male infants
(2) presents during the first few days of life
(3) presents with vomiting, dehydration, and malnutrition
(4) resolves spontaneously if symptomatic medical management is promptly instituted

265. Which of the following conditions can be considered characteristic of congenital megacolon (Hirschsprung's disease)?

(1) Absence of ganglion cells from the myenteric plexus
(2) Constipation
(3) Intestinal distension
(4) Hematemesis

266. Which of the following conditions may be associated with acute gastric ulceration?

(1) Extensive burns
(2) Cerebrovascular accidents
(3) Corticosteroid therapy
(4) Excessive alcohol intake

267. The diarrhea associated with the Zollinger-Ellison syndrome may be due to

(1) gastric hypersecretion
(2) increased intestinal motility
(3) malabsorption syndrome
(4) excessive 5-hydroxytryptamine

268. Lesions in the stomach that are associated with a higher than normal rate of development of gastric cancer include

(1) achlorhydria
(2) pernicious anemia
(3) atrophic gastritis
(4) adenomatous polyps

269. Which of the following conditions may produce intestinal mucosal ulceration?

(1) Uremia
(2) Typhoid enteritis
(3) Ulcerative colitis
(4) Staphylococcal colitis

270. Findings characteristic of celiac disease include

(1) relationship to gluten in the diet
(2) lymphangiectasia in the intestinal mucosa
(3) loss of villi in the small intestine
(4) reversibility with folic acid therapy

271. Which of the following statements correctly characterize the colonic lesion shown below?

(1) The prevalence is highest in people under 50 years of age
(2) The lesions are more common in women
(3) Lesions occur most frequently in the ascending and transverse segments of the colon
(4) The lesions occur more commonly in the colon than in other portions of the gastrointestinal tract

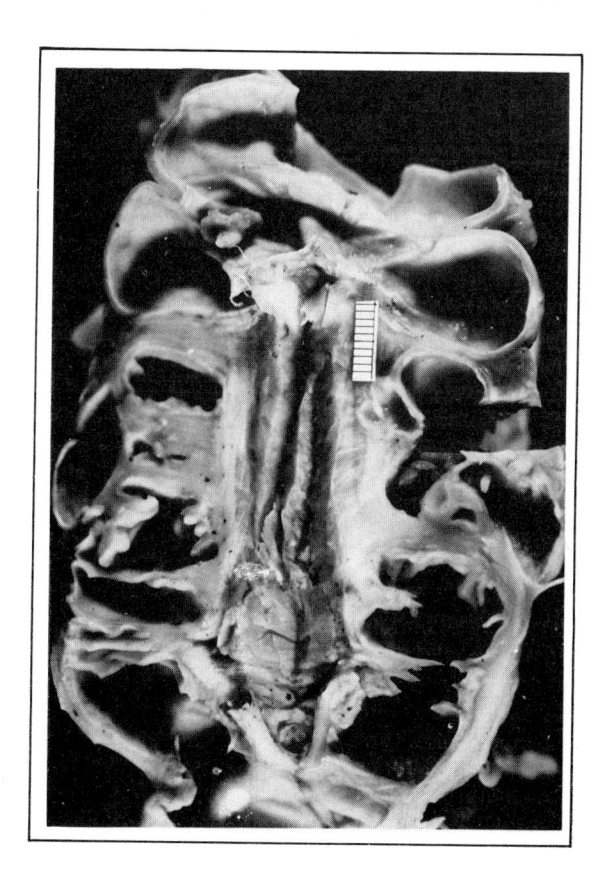

SUMMARY OF DIRECTIONS

A	B	C	D	E
1, 2, 3 only	1, 3 only	2, 4 only	4 only	All are correct

272. Which of the following conditions are thought to play a role in the pathogenesis of diverticulosis?

(1) Bacterial infection
(2) Vascular insufficiency
(3) Absence of myenteric plexus
(4) Increased intraluminal pressure

273. Which of the following conditions may be difficult to distinguish clinically from acute appendicitis?

(1) Mesenteric lymphadenitis
(2) Ruptured ovarian follicle
(3) Acute salpingitis
(4) Regional enteritis

274. Conditions causing or exacerbating hemorrhoids include

(1) cirrhosis of the liver with portal hypertension
(2) carcinoma of the rectum
(3) pregnancy
(4) chronic constipation

275. Jaundice may be produced by

(1) increased rate of bilirubin production
(2) decreased uptake in liver cells
(3) derangements in conjugation with glucuronide
(4) impaired secretion into the biliary tract

276. Extrahepatic biliary obstruction may

(1) cause conjugated hyperbilirubinemia
(2) lead to cirrhosis
(3) be confused clinically with viral hepatitis
(4) be due to choledocholithiasis

277. Central necrosis of the liver may be caused by

(1) chloroform
(2) carbon tetrachloride
(3) cardiac failure
(4) eclampsia

278. Which of the following findings characterize chronic passive congestion of the liver?

(1) Fibrosis about central veins
(2) Mottling of the surface
(3) Widening of the sinusoids
(4) Bile infarcts

279. A patient with ascending cholangitis, as illustrated below, probably also has

(1) common duct obstruction
(2) cholelithiasis
(3) gram-negative bacteremia
(4) cholestasis

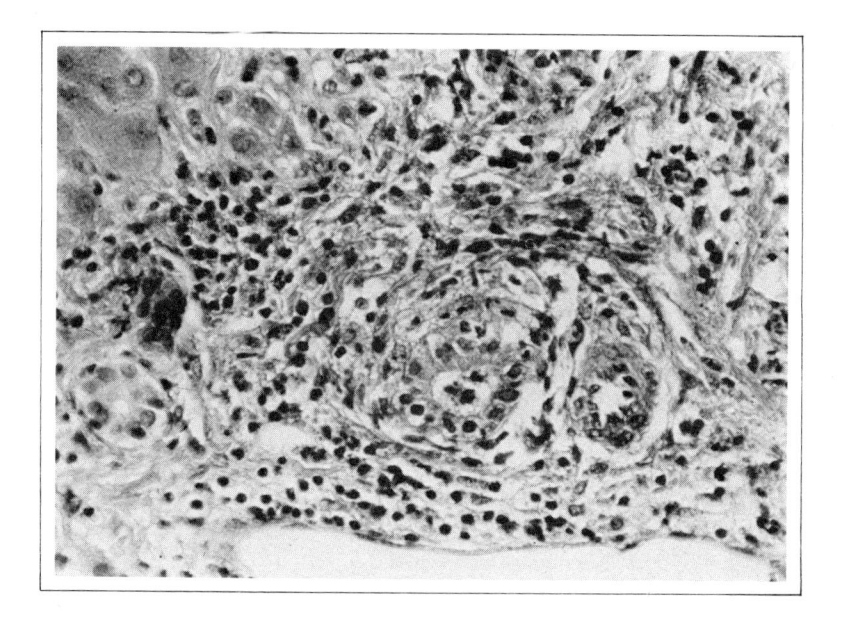

280. Common findings associated with infectious viral hepatitis include

(1) fever
(2) a short incubation period
(3) a four to six week course
(4) mild liver disturbances

281. Hepatic granulomas may be seen in

(1) sarcoidosis
(2) tuberculosis
(3) histoplasmosis
(4) Hodgkin's disease

282. Features necessary for the diagnosis of cirrhosis of the liver include

(1) nodular hepatic regeneration
(2) bile duct proliferation
(3) fibrosis
(4) fatty change

SUMMARY OF DIRECTIONS				
A	B	C	D	E
1, 2, 3 only	1, 3 only	2, 4 only	4 only	All are correct

283. Finely nodular (micronodular) cirrhosis as pictured below, is usually associated with

(1) massive hepatic necrosis
(2) increased fat within hepatocytes
(3) viral hepatitis
(4) alcohol abuse

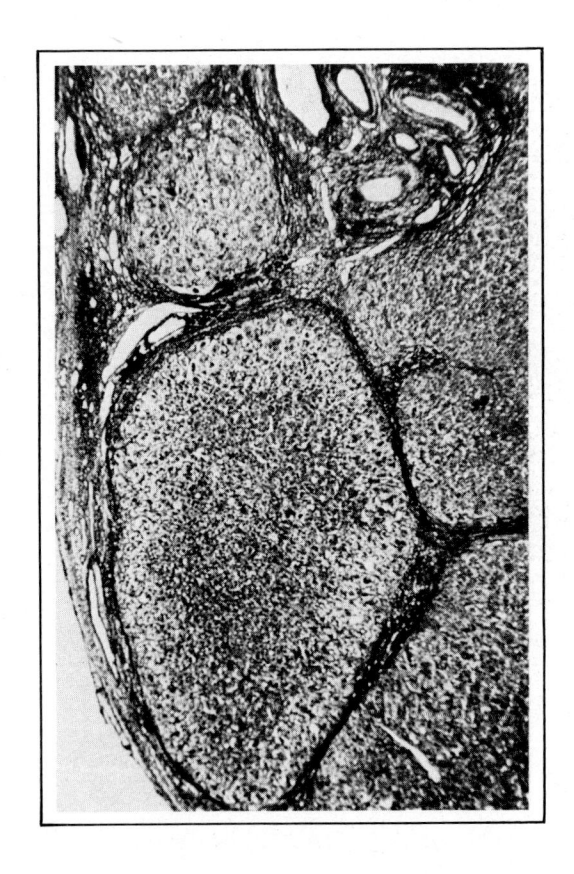

DIRECTIONS: The groups of questions in this section consist of four lettered headings followed by several numbered items. For each numbered item choose the **one** lettered heading with which it is **most** closely associated. Each lettered heading may be used once, more than once, or not at all.

Questions 284-286
Match the following.

(A) Hyperplastic (adenomatous) polyp
(B) Papillary (villous) adenoma
(C) Both
(D) Neither

284. Most common polypoid lesion of the stomach

285. Histologic evidence of cellular atypia and malignant transformation is common

286. Lesions are frequently larger than 2 cm in diameter

Questions 287-290
Match the following.

(A) Primary biliary cirrhosis
(B) Laennec's cirrhosis
(C) Both
(D) Neither

287. Associated with alcohol abuse

288. Bile duct proliferation

289. Xanthomas of skin and ulcerative colitis

290. Equal sex incidence

Endocrine System

DIRECTIONS: Each question below contains five suggested answers. Choose the **one best** response to each question.

291. The most common etiologic factor in Cushing's syndrome is

(A) adrenal adenoma
(B) bilateral adrenal hyperplasia
(C) adrenal carcinoma
(D) ectopic adrenal tissue
(E) hypercorticism secondary to nonendocrine malignant tumors

292. Symmetrical bilateral calcification of basal ganglia may be seen in

(A) hypoparathyroidism
(B) idiopathic parkinsonism
(C) kernicterus
(D) ochronosis
(E) vitamin D intoxication

293. The combination of cystic bone lesions, precocious puberty, and patchy skin pigmentation is known as

(A) Albright's syndrome
(B) Letterer-Siwe disease
(C) Asherman's syndrome
(D) Morquio's disease
(E) Schaumann's disease

294. Hyalinization of the islets of the pancreas in a 30-year-old patient is most commonly found in

(A) pancreatic duct obstruction
(B) cystic fibrosis
(C) carcinoma
(D) chronic renal failure
(E) diabetes mellitus

295. Which thyroid lesion is most likely to cause hyperthyroidism?

(A) Papillary carcinoma
(B) Diffuse hyperplasia (Graves' disease)
(C) Riedel's struma
(D) Fetal adenoma
(E) Colloid goiter

296. A helpful sign in distinguishing between primary and secondary adrenal insufficiency is

(A) temporal blindness
(B) skin pigmentation
(C) bone pain
(D) dystrophic calcifications
(E) weight loss

297. The piece of tissue shown below (low power view) was probably removed from a

(A) normal thyroid gland
(B) colloid storage goiter
(C) patient with Graves' disease
(D) patient with Riedel's struma
(E) patient with Hashimoto's thyroiditis

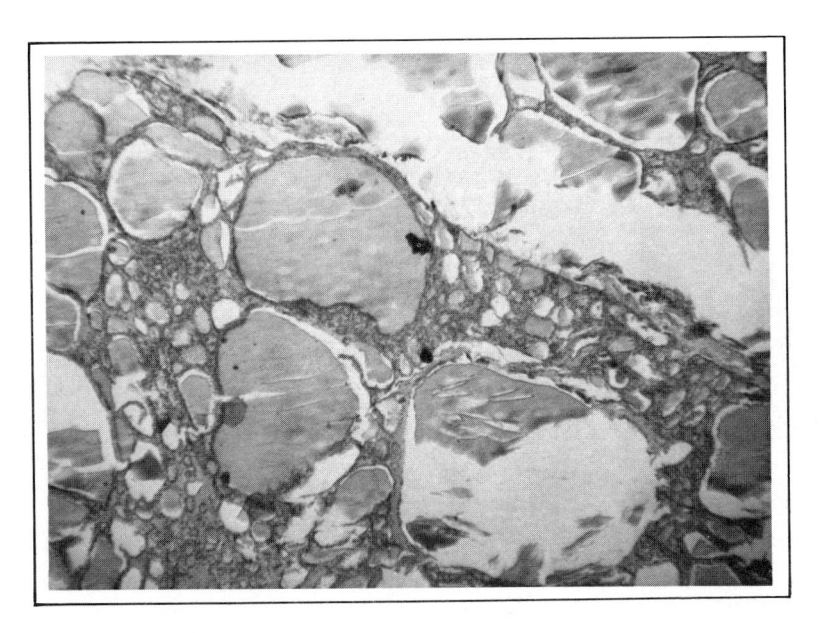

298. A partially calcified cystic lesion in the region of the sella turcica is probably

(A) brain abscess
(B) craniopharyngioma
(C) ependymoma
(D) cavernous sinus thrombosis
(E) metastatic carcinoma

299. Pituitary infarction is most likely to be caused by

(A) renal failure
(B) postpartum hemorrhage
(C) cirrhosis
(D) atherosclerosis
(E) hypertension

300. Secondary hyperparathyroidism may be caused by

(A) chronic renal insufficiency
(B) Hashimoto's thyroiditis
(C) pituitary hyperplasia
(D) alcoholic hepatitis
(E) acute pancreatitis

301. Medullary carcinoma of the thyroid is thought to arise from

(A) acinar cells
(B) lymphocytes
(C) C cells (parafollicular cells)
(D) stromal fibroblasts
(E) endothelial cells

302. Hemorrhagic adrenal necrosis classically occurs as a result of infection with

(A) coxsackievirus
(B) *Neisseria meningitidis*
(C) *Treponema pallidum*
(D) *Candida albicans*
(E) *Streptococcus*

303. The histamine vasopressor test may be used to diagnose

(A) asthma
(B) chromophobe adenoma
(C) pheochromocytoma
(D) prostatic carcinoma
(E) Cushing's syndrome

304. In a patient with acromegaly, the most common pituitary tumor is a

(A) basophilic adenoma
(B) craniopharyngeoma
(C) acidophilic adenoma
(D) teratoma
(E) chromophobe adenoma

305. Tumors of the thymus (thymomas) occur in a significant proportion of patients with

(A) cystic fibrosis
(B) myasthenia gravis
(C) Marfan's syndrome
(D) multiple myeloma
(E) bronchogenic carcinoma

306. Which of the following signs is NOT characteristic of Cushing's syndrome?

(A) Moon face
(B) Abdominal stria
(C) Hypotension
(D) Poor muscle development
(E) Osteoporosis

DIRECTIONS: Each question below contains four suggested answers of which **one** or **more** is correct. Choose the answer

A	if	1, 2, and 3	are correct
B	if	1 and 3	are correct
C	if	2 and 4	are correct
D	if	4	is correct
E	if	1, 2, 3, and 4	are correct

307. Which of the following renal lesions are more common in patients with diabetes mellitus than in the general population?

(1) Nodular glomerulosclerosis
(2) Hyaline arteriolosclerosis of the efferent renal arterioles
(3) Glycogen nephrosis
(4) Necrotizing papillitis

308. Chronic adrenal insufficiency may be caused by

(1) adrenal atrophy
(2) tuberculosis
(3) amyloidosis
(4) carcinomatosis

309. Radiologic evidence of hyperparathyroidism includes

(1) erosion of the distal clavicle
(2) loss of the lamina dura about the teeth
(3) "brown tumors" of bone
(4) bone cysts

DIRECTIONS: The groups of questions in this section consist of four or five lettered headings followed by several numbered items. For each numbered item choose the **one** lettered heading with which it it **most.** closely associated. Each lettered heading may be used once, more than once, or not at all.

Questions 310-313
For each tumor, choose the sign with which it is most likely to be associated.

(A) Hypoglycemia
(B) Polycythemia
(C) Cushing's syndrome
(D) Monoclonal gammopathy
(E) Malignant hypertension

310. Adenoma of islets of Langerhans

311. Retroperitoneal fibrosarcoma

312. Renal cell carcinoma

313. Adrenal cortical adenoma

Questions 314-317
Match the following.

(A) Papillary carcinoma of thyroid gland
(B) Medullary carcinoma of thyroid gland
(C) Both
(D) Neither

314. Metastases occur most frequently in adjacent lymph nodes of the neck

315. Associated with psammoma bodies

316. Association with other endocrine tumors

317. Rapidly growing, focally infiltrative growth with a poor prognosis

Genitourinary System

DIRECTIONS: Each question below contains five suggested answers. Choose the **one best** response to each question.

318. A large abdominal mass arising from the kidney of a child is most likely to be a

(A) neuroblastoma
(B) renal cortical adenoma
(C) Wilms' tumor
(D) histiocytic lymphoma
(E) medullary sponge kidney

319. Primary hyperoxaluria frequently leads to renal failure and death due to

(A) calcium oxalate deposits
(B) oxalic acid deficiency
(C) impairment of the degradation of oxalic acid
(D) severe acidosis by oxalic acid
(E) blockage of the conversion of glycolic acid to glyoxylic acid

320. The most common underlying renal disease in renal vein thrombosis is

(A) chronic pyelonephritis
(B) chronic glomerulonephritis
(C) gouty nephropathy
(D) renal amyloidosis
(E) polycystic kidneys

321. A linear pattern of immunoglobulin deposition along the glomerular basement membrane which can be demonstrated by immunofluorescence is typical of

(A) lupus nephritis
(B) diabetic glomerulopathy
(C) Goodpasture's syndrome
(D) Goldblatt's kidney
(E) renal vein thrombosis

322. What is the correct treatment for a patient with hypertension secondary to unilateral renal artery stenosis, when the contralateral kidney shows severe arteriolonephrosclerosis?

(A) Ureteral reimplantation
(B) Removal of the kidney supplied by the stenotic artery
(C) Repair of the renal artery stenosis and ipsilateral nephrectomy
(D) Repair of the renal artery stenosis and contralateral nephrectomy
(E) Medical management

323. Marked glomerular basement membrane thickening, as shown below, may be seen in all of the following conditions EXCEPT

(A) lupus nephritis
(B) membranous glomerulonephritis
(C) diabetes mellitus
(D) acute pyelonephritis
(E) renal vein thrombosis

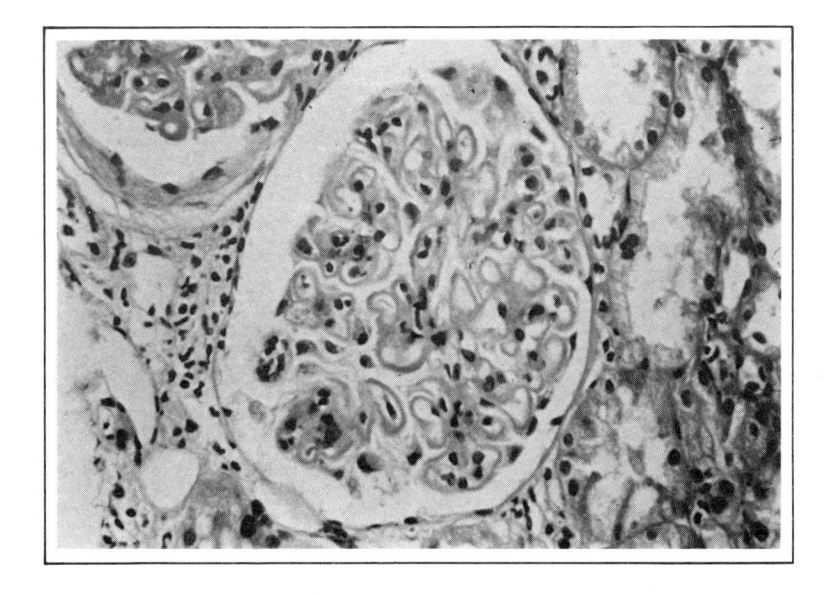

324. The presence of one normal kidney and one shrunken kidney with coarse cortical scars and deformity of the pelvis and calyces is most compatible with a diagnosis of

(A) chronic glomerulonephritis
(B) amyloidosis
(C) chronic pyelonephritis
(D) renal artery stenosis
(E) necrotizing papillitis

325. The classic presenting complaint of a patient with epithelial bladder carcinoma is

(A) abdominal pain referred to the suprapubic region
(B) painless hematuria
(C) dysuria
(D) retention with painful overflow
(E) frequency with oliguria

326. The most common site of carcinoma in adult males is the

(A) esophagus
(B) stomach
(C) intestine
(D) lung
(E) prostate

327. Poststreptococcal glomerulonephritis is usually associated with infection by which type of group A streptococci?

(A) Type 4
(B) Type 12
(C) Type 18
(D) Type 25
(E) No specific type

328. A 40-year-old woman was diagnosed as having tuberculosis. She complained of severe lower abdominal pain. The most likely region of involvement would be the

(A) endocervix
(B) ovary
(C) uterine wall
(D) fallopian tube
(E) vaginal mucosa

329. Most ectopic pregnancies occur within the

(A) intrauterine portion of the fallopian tubes
(B) tubular portion of the fallopian tubes
(C) ovarian fimbria
(D) ovary
(E) abdominal cavity

330. Endometrial glands and stroma deep within the myometrium are found in

(A) adenomyosis
(B) invasive adenocarcinoma of the uterus
(C) endometriosis
(D) choriocarcinoma
(E) metastatic carcinoma

331. The cell type most specifically associated with primary chronic endometritis is

(A) neutrophil
(B) lymphocyte
(C) plasma cell
(D) histiocyte
(E) eosinophil

332. Invasive squamous carcinoma of the cervix may be associated with all of the following EXCEPT

(A) carcinoma in situ
(B) age at onset of sexual intercourse
(C) estrogen administration
(D) prostitution
(E) severe squamous dysplasia

333. Cystic structures frequently appear in all of the following ovarian lesions EXCEPT

(A) hilar cell tumor
(B) adenofibroma
(C) Brenner tumor
(D) entodermal sinus tumor
(E) serous cystadenoma

334. The occasional finding of intestinal mucosa and intestinal enzymes (such as lipase, trypsin, amylase, and sucrase) in mucinous cystadenomas of the ovary suggests that the

(A) cystadenomas are usually metastatic colon carcinomas
(B) cystadenomas may arise from teratomas
(C) cystadenomas should be treated with estrogens
(D) cystadenomas have metastasized to the intestine
(E) patient has virilization

335. The ovarian lesion illustrated below is

(A) chronic salpingitis
(B) an ectopic pregnancy
(C) a granulosa cell tumor
(D) a cystic teratoma
(E) metastatic squamous cell carcinoma

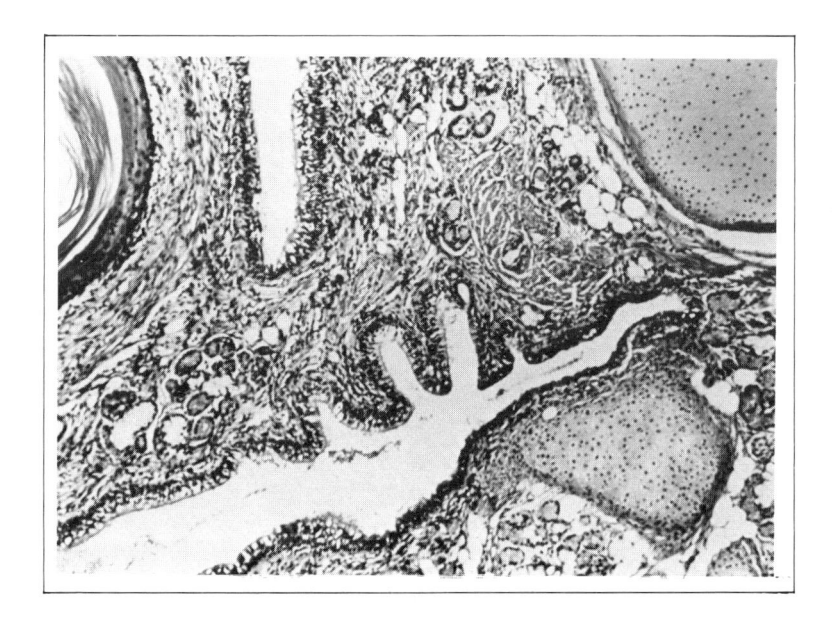

336. Ovarian cystadenomas or cystadenocarcinomas (serous or mucinous)

(A) always produce androgens
(B) seldom are bilateral
(C) can be papillary
(D) usually occur during pregnancy
(E) are extremely rare

337. Metastatic, mucin-producing, signet-ring cancer cells in the ovary most frequently come from

(A) intestinal carcinoma
(B) malignant melanoma
(C) astrocytoma
(D) histiocytic lymphoma
(E) endometrial carcinoma

338. The patient whose testicular biopsy is illustrated below would have been most likely to complain to his physician of

(A) hematuria
(B) testicular pain
(C) testicular enlargement
(D) infertility
(E) hypertension

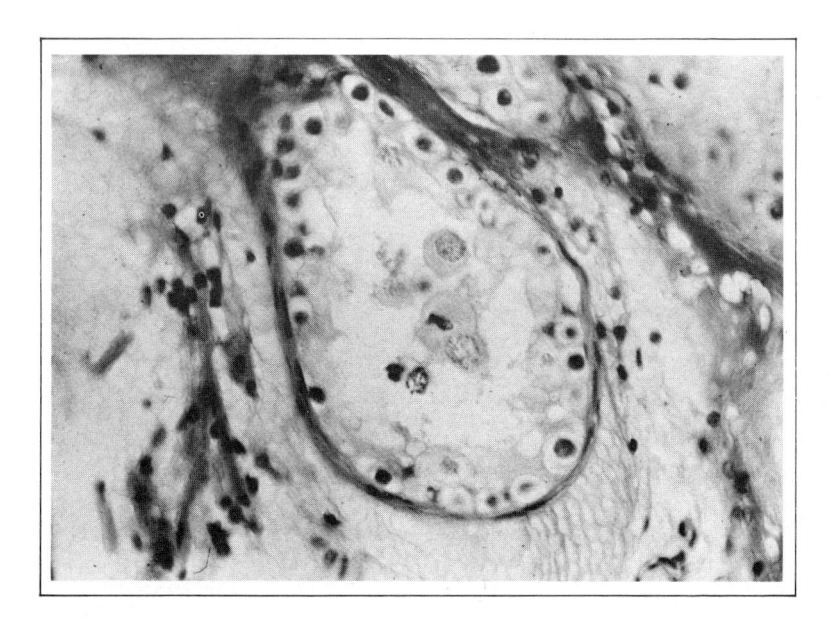

339. In men between the age of 25 and 35 years, the most common cancer is

(A) Hodgkin's lymphoma
(B) non-Hodgkin's lymphoma
(C) chronic myelogenous leukemia
(D) osteogenic sarcoma
(E) germ cell tumors

340. Which of the following testicular tumors most often presents as a malignant lesion?

(A) Teratoma
(B) Seminoma
(C) Interstitial cell tumor
(D) Adenomatoid tumor
(E) Leydig cell tumor

341. Carcinoma of the prostate usually arises

(A) in the median lobe
(B) in the posterior lobe
(C) in the anterior lobe
(D) in either of the two lateral lobes
(E) with equal distribution among the lobes

DIRECTIONS: Each question below contains four suggested answers of which **one** or **more** is correct. Choose the answer

A	if	1, 2, and 3	are correct
B	if	1 and 3	are correct
C	if	2 and 4	are correct
D	if	4	is correct
E	if	1, 2, 3, and 4	are correct

342. Necrotizing papillitis may be seen in patients with

(1) diabetes mellitus
(2) sickle cell anemia
(3) phenacetin nephropathy
(4) Wilson's disease

343. Acute pyelonephritis

(1) spares the renal tubules
(2) is usually caused by gram-negative bacteria
(3) leads to urinary tract obstruction
(4) may follow urinary tract instrumentation

344. Acute poststreptococcal glomerulonephritis usually

(1) affects children
(2) follows a streptococcal infection by more than six months
(3) is accompanied by decreased serum complement
(4) leads to chronic renal failure

345. The nephrotic syndrome

(1) may occur with renal vein thrombosis
(2) is characterized by decreased serum lipid levels
(3) may occur in membranous glomerulonephritis
(4) usually presents with hematuria

346. Which of the following renal diseases may cause hypertension?

(1) Renal artery arteriosclerosis
(2) Hydronephrosis
(3) Fibromuscular dysplasia of the renal artery
(4) Pyelonephritis

347. Which of the following conditions result in grossly shrunken kidneys?

(1) Acute renal failure following hypovolemic shock
(2) Arteriolar nephrosclerosis
(3) Amyloidosis
(4) Chronic glomerulonephritis

Question 348-350

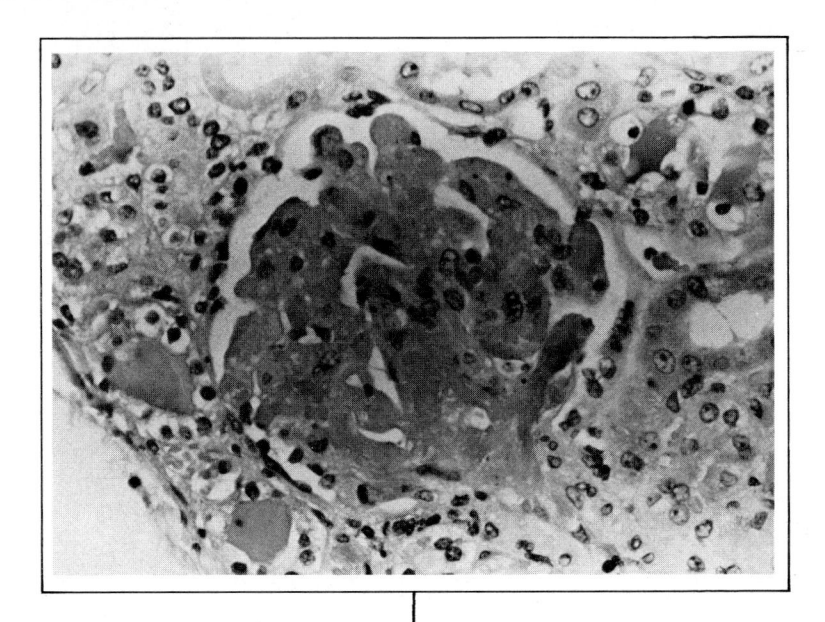

348. The process of glomerular fibrin deposition, shown above, in a 2-year-old child with a history of acute gastroenteritis followed by acute glomerulonephritis, severe Coombs'-negative hemolytic anemia, and renal failure, is consistent with a diagnosis of

(1) lupus erythematosus
(2) acute poststreptococcal glomerulonephritis
(3) lipoid nephrosis
(4) hemolytic uremic syndrome

349. Which of the following statements concerning the pathologic process described above, in young children, are true?

(1) Patients with severe, acute disease with long periods of oliguria, frequently die or sustain permanent renal damage
(2) There is evidence to suggest an infectious etiology
(3) The disease includes a spectrum ranging from focal or partial glomerular necrosis to cortical necrosis
(4) Steroids and anticoagulation therapy have been successful in treating a majority of cases

350. Other renal diseases in which fibrin thrombi play a prominent role include

(1) lipoid nephrosis
(2) membranous glomerulopathy
(3) diabetes mellitus
(4) anaphylactoid nephritis (Henoch-Schönlein purpura)

351. The hyalinized glomeruli demonstrated in the photomicrograph of renal cortex shown below could result from

(1) arteriolar nephrosclerosis
(2) chronic pyelonephritis
(3) chronic glomerulonephritis
(4) chronic rejection reaction

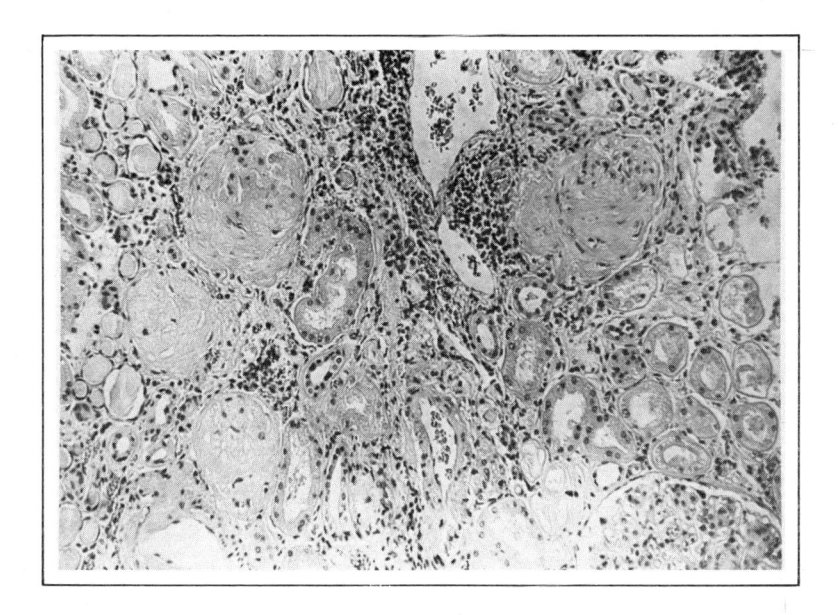

352. Type I polycystic kidney disease is

(1) rarely seen in adults
(2) a disease with numerous renal cysts that arise from collecting tubules
(3) always bilateral
(4) generally compatible with a life span of several decades as long as the cysts do not encroach on and compromise the residual renal function

SUMMARY OF DIRECTIONS

A	B	C	D	E
1, 2, 3 only	1, 3 only	2, 4 only	4 only	All are correct

Questions 353-354

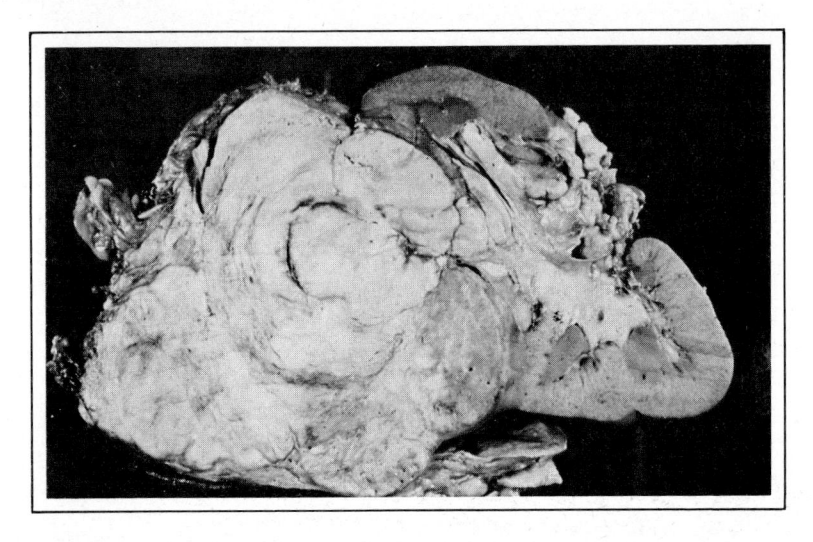

353. The primary renal carcinoma shown above

(1) may be bright yellow
(2) is a squamous or papillary carcinoma
(3) invades the renal veins
(4) probably secretes ACTH

354. The renal cell carcinoma illustrated above may

(1) metastasize to bone
(2) produce hypercalcemia
(3) produce polycythemia
(4) contain glycogen

355. Carcinoma of the prostate tends to

(1) occur most often in the lateral lobes of the gland
(2) exhibit perineural invasion
(3) be estrogen dependent
(4) cause elevation of the serum acid phosphatase

356. Papillary carcinoma of the bladder may

(1) contain transitional epithelium
(2) be related to smoking
(3) recur following excision
(4) cause hematuria

357. The botryoid (grapelike) neoplasm, shown below, arising in the urinary bladder

(1) may contain malignant rhabdomyoblasts
(2) is most likely to be a papillary carcinoma
(3) may also arise in the vagina
(4) has a good prognosis

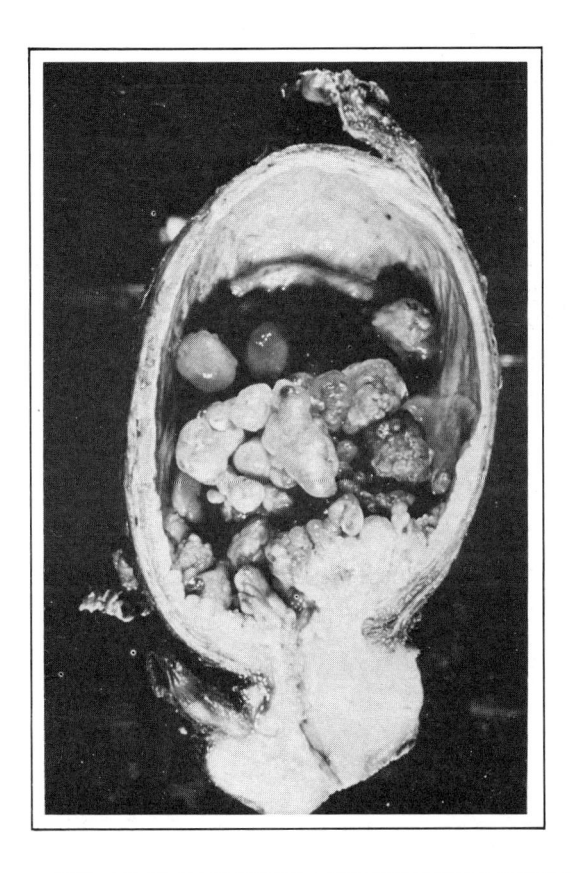

SUMMARY OF DIRECTIONS

A	B	C	D	E
1, 2, 3 only	1, 3 only	2, 4 only	4 only	All are correct

83

Questions 358-359

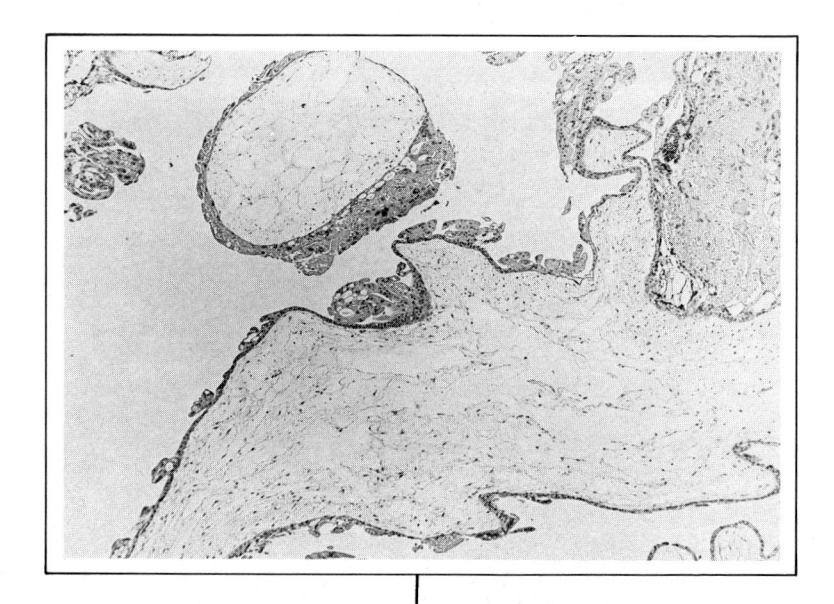

358. Hydatidiform swelling of the type illustrated in the photomicrograph above can occur

(1) at the margins of normal placentas where fetal circulation is impaired
(2) in otherwise normal placentas with focal, villous, vascular anomalies
(3) in chorionic villi of blighted ova
(4) in choriocarcinoma

359. Microscopic features of hydatidiform moles include

(1) variation in the degree of trophoblastic proliferation and cellular atypia
(2) invasion of the myometrium
(3) avascularity of the villous stalk
(4) remnants of fetal tissue

SUMMARY OF DIRECTIONS				
A	B	C	D	E
1, 2, 3 only	1, 3 only	2, 4 only	4 only	All are correct

360. The well-differentiated, superficial squamous cells shown below were the predominant cell type seen is a Papanicolaou smear of the lateral vaginal wall. The patient probably is

(1) postmenopausal
(2) being treated for cervical carcinoma
(3) receiving androgens
(4) premenopausal

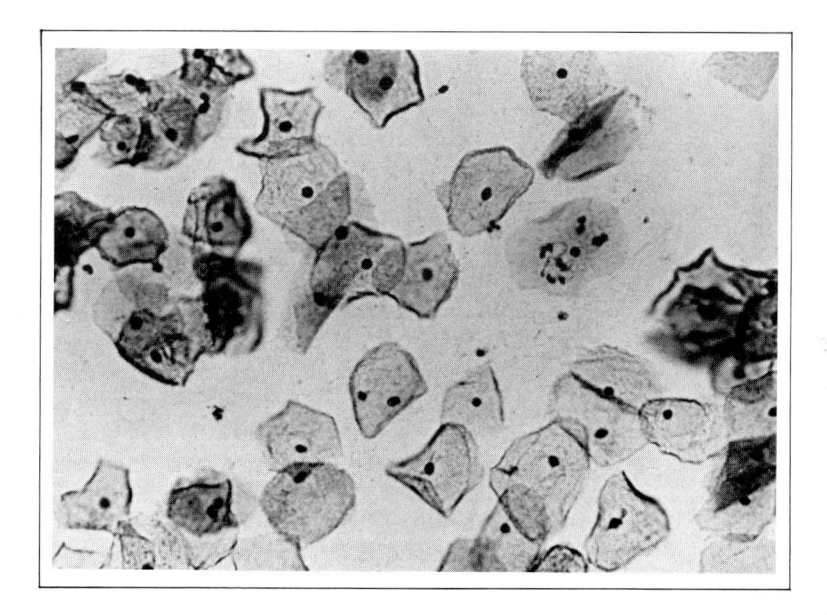

361. Endometriosis

(1) is a malignant lesion
(2) may involve the ovaries
(3) can be diagnosed on Pap smear
(4) can undergo cyclic menstrual changes with periodic bleeding

362. Cystic hyperplasia of the endometrium

(1) occurs at, or just before, menopause
(2) occurs in association with increased estrogen administration or production
(3) usually results in excessive uterine bleeding
(4) is associated with secretory cells lining the cystically dilated glands

363. Suppurative salpingitis may

(1) be caused by gonococci
(2) lead to a tubo-ovarian abscess
(3) cause sterility
(4) be a typical manifestation of primary syphilis

364. Which of the following diseases occur more commonly than normal in the children of women who received diethylstilbestrol during pregnancy?

(1) Vaginal adenosis
(2) Sarcoma botryoides
(3) Vaginal adenocarcinoma
(4) Breast carcinoma

365. Choriocarcinoma of the uterus

(1) is a malignancy of trophoblastic cells
(2) responds poorly to chemotherapy
(3) may arise in a hydatidiform mole
(4) never follows a normal pregnancy

366. Carcinoma of the endometrium appears to be more frequent in patients with

(1) obesity
(2) diabetes mellitus
(3) hypertension
(4) breast carcinoma

367. Uterine leiomyomas

(1) never become calcified
(2) may increase in size during pregnancy
(3) frequently metastasize
(4) are common tumors

SUMMARY OF DIRECTIONS

A	B	C	D	E
1, 2, 3 only	1, 3 only	2, 4 only	4 only	All are correct

368. Ovarian neoplasms of germ cell origin include

(1) serous cystadenoma
(2) thecoma
(3) Brenner tumor
(4) dysgerminoma

369. A granulosa cell tumor of the ovary may produce excess estrogen and cause

(1) menstrual irregularities
(2) endometrial hyperplasia
(3) precocious puberty
(4) uterine enlargement

370. Ascites and pleural effusion in a woman with a primary ovarian neoplasm

(1) always means that the tumor has metastasized and is thus inoperable
(2) is strong presumptive evidence that a granulosa cell tumor is present in an ovary
(3) should be treated with intrapleural administration of methotrexate and actinomycin D
(4) may occur with a benign ovarian fibroma

371. Which of the following are considered premalignant lesions in the penis?

(1) Leukoplakia
(2) Erythroplasia of Queyrat
(3) Bowen's disease
(4) Phimosis

372. Carcinoma of the prostate

(1) may increase alkaline phosphatase
(2) may increase acid phosphatase
(3) most often produces osteoblastic metastases
(4) most often presents as hematuria

373. Mumps orchitis generally

(1) is bilateral
(2) results in sterility
(3) occurs simultaneously with parotid swelling
(4) occurs in adults

DIRECTIONS: The groups of questions in this section consist of four or five lettered headings followed by several numbered items. For each numbered item choose the **one** lettered heading with which it is **most** closely associated. Each lettered heading may be used once, more than once, or not at all.

Questions 374-378

For each structure, identify its location by letter in the electron micrograph of a renal glomerulus shown below.

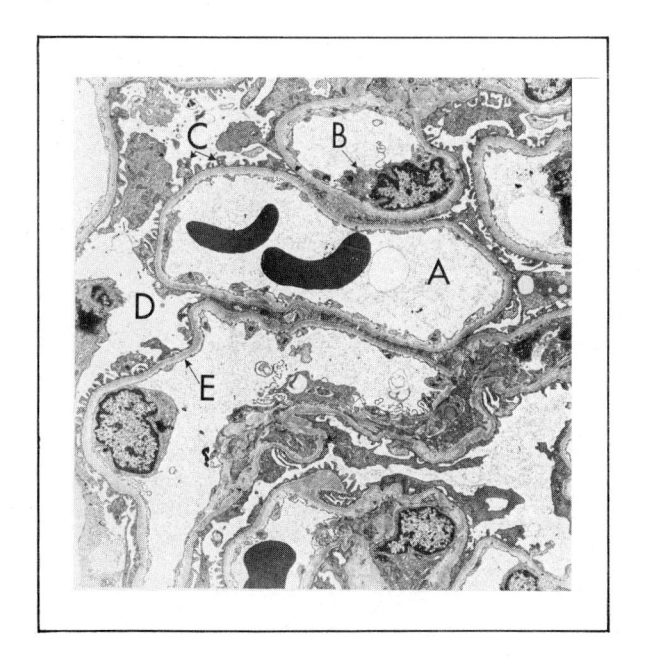

374. Basement membrane

375. Endothelial cell

376. Epithelial cell foot processes

377. Capillary lumen

378. Bowman's space

Questions 379-381
For each pathologic finding, choose the etiologic condition with which it is most likely to be associated.

(A) Disseminated intravascular coagulation
(B) Hyperuricemia
(C) Vegetative endocarditis
(D) Hypersplenism
(E) Constrictive pericarditis

379. Hydronephrosis

380. Diffuse cortical necrosis

381. Focal renal infarction

Questions 382-384
For each pathologic finding, choose the disease in which it is most characteristic.

(A) Malignant hypertension
(B) Systemic lupus erythematosus
(C) Chronic thyroiditis
(D) Addison's disease
(E) Diabetes mellitus

382. Hyperplastic arteriolar nephrosclerosis

383. Nodular intercapillary glomerulosclerosis

384. Necrotizing papillitis

Questions 385-388
Match the following.

(A) Nephroblastoma
(B) Neuroblastoma
(C) Both
(D) Neither

385. Malignant tumor capable of metastasis

386. Metastases characteristically found in bones

387. Histologic sections may show embryonal rhabdomyoblasts (primitive skeletal muscle)

388. Lesions usually arise in adolescents

Nervous System

DIRECTIONS: Each question below contains five suggested answers. Choose the **one best** response to each question.

389. Herpes zoster usually

(A) causes smallpox
(B) follows the distribution of nerves
(C) causes a fatal disease
(D) does not infect humans
(E) causes a painless infection

390. Toxoplasmosis causes

(A) severe symptoms in adults
(B) muscle lesions
(C) encephalitis in the newborn
(D) sexual abnormalities
(E) dermatologic scars

391. Subdural effusion may occur in infants with any form of meningitis, but is most commonly seen in connection with meningitis due to

(A) streptococci
(B) staphylococci
(C) pneumococci
(D) *Hemophilus influenzae*
(E) tubercle bacilli

392. In poliomyelitis, the pathologic findings principally involve the

(A) anterior horn cells
(B) cerebellum
(C) thalamus
(D) muscle fibers of the leg
(E) caudate nucleus

393. Ganglioside lipidosis is a fatal disease which classically first becomes evident in four- to six-month-old children. It is characterized by

(A) blindness, associated with a cherry-red spot in the retina
(B) enlargement and coloration of the tonsils
(C) enlargement of the liver and spleen
(D) the appearance of tuberous xanthomas
(E) dark coloration of the urine

394. Which of the following central nervous system cell populations is the most rapidly affected by ischemia?

(A) Axis cylinders
(B) Nerve cell bodies
(C) Astrocytes
(D) Microglia
(E) Oligodendroglia

395. The most common lesion in Wernicke's encephalopathy is found in the

(A) substantia nigra
(B) motor cortex
(C) mamillary bodies
(D) dentate nucleus
(E) cranial nerve nuclei

396. A hypertensive patient who develops a "stroke" probably has

(A) a dural sinus thrombosis
(B) ruptured an aneurysm
(C) suffered an intracerebral hemorrhage
(D) developed a cerebral infarct
(E) compressed his basilar artery

397. The most common region of spontaneous intracranial hemorrhage is the

(A) medullar
(B) meninges
(C) cerebral hemispheres
(D) pons
(E) cerebellum

398. Pseudopalisading, necrosis, endoneurial proliferation, hypercellularity, and nuclear atypicality are most characteristic of which of the following tumors?

(A) Schwannoma
(B) Medulloblastoma
(C) Oligodendroglioma
(D) Glioblastoma multiforme
(E) Ependymoma

399. Astrocytomas are the

(A) least invasive gliomas
(B) most common form of glioma
(C) least severe form of glioma
(D) only glial type of tumor in humans
(E) most rapidly growing gliomas

400. Which of the following tumors is most likely to "seed" through the nervous system?

(A) Medulloblastoma
(B) Oligodendroglioma
(C) Pinealoma
(D) Choroid plexus papilloma
(E) Meningioma

401. Which of the following brain tumors is noted for its radiosensitivity?

(A) Astrocytoma
(B) Glioblastoma multiforme
(C) Meningioma
(D) Ependymoma
(E) Medulloblastoma

402. Which of the following is NOT a tumor of the peripheral nervous system cells?

(A) Neuroma
(B) Schwannoma
(C) Neurilemoma
(D) Neurofibroma
(E) Neuroblastoma

403. The form of motor neuron disease in which there is weakness and atrophy of muscles, without corticospinal tract dysfunction, is known as

(A) amyotrophic lateral sclerosis
(B) progressive muscular atrophy
(C) Werdnig-Hoffmann syndrome
(D) primary lateral sclerosis
(E) Charcot-Marie-Tooth disease

404. A retinoblastoma is most similar to a

(A) fibroma
(B) pheochromocytoma
(C) neuroblastoma
(D) astrocytoma
(E) angioma

DIRECTIONS: Each question below contains four suggested answers of which **one** or **more** is correct. Choose the answer

A	if	1, 2, and 3	are correct
B	if	1 and 3	are correct
C	if	2 and 4	are correct
D	if	4	is correct
E	if	1, 2, 3, and 4	are correct

405. Meningiomas

(1) constitute 15 percent of all brain tumors
(2) are more common in children than adults
(3) are more common in women than men
(4) usually are not amenable to surgical therapy

406. Intracerebral hemorrhage may be secondary to

(1) hypertensive cerebral vascular disease
(2) trauma
(3) rupture of an aneurysm
(4) blood dyscrasia

407. Important causes of cerebral infarction include

(1) arteriosclerotic vascular disease
(2) acute lead poisoning
(3) cerebral embolization
(4) equine encephalitis

408. Hypertensive hemorrhage is common in which of the following anatomic sites?

(1) Internal capsule-basal ganglia
(2) Pons
(3) Cerebellum
(4) Medulla

409. Hydrocephalus may be caused by

(1) absence of the choroid plexus
(2) overproduction of cerebrospinal fluid
(3) thrombosis of the foramen of Winslow
(4) stenosis of the aqueduct of Sylvius

410. Development of bilirubin encephalopathy depends upon the

(1) plasma albumin level
(2) type of hyperbilirubinemia
(3) status of acid-base balance
(4) degree of hyperbilirubinemia

411. In multiple neuritis

(1) some peripheral nerves are totally destroyed
(2) the distribution of lesions is often unilateral
(3) fasciculations are characteristic
(4) distal extremities are greatly affected

412. Which of the following characterize idiopathic parkinsonism?

(1) Cerebral edema
(2) Depigmentation and loss of neurons in the substantia nigra
(3) Neurofibrillary tangles
(4) Lewy bodies

413. The process of primary demyelination is fundamental to

(1) Pelizaeus-Merzbacher disease
(2) Krabbe's disease
(3) Schilder's disease
(4) metachromatic leukodystrophy

414. Which of the following diseases are classified as demyelinating?

(1) Multiple sclerosis
(2) Arnold-Chiari syndrome
(3) Postinfectious encephalomyelitis
(4) Myasthenia gravis

415. The characteristic abnormalities seen in patients with Refsum's disease include

(1) polyneuritis
(2) ichthyosis
(3) retinopathy
(4) anosmia

416. Tabes dorsalis causes

(1) bilateral degeneration of dorsal nerve roots
(2) a positive Romberg sign
(3) severe impairment of vibratory sense
(4) progressive sensitivity to pain

417. Amyotrophic lateral sclerosis

(1) is not always fatal
(2) causes sensory loss, secondary to dorsal nerve root involvement
(3) produces spasticity of all affected muscles
(4) causes weakness, atrophy, and fasciculations of hand muscles

418. Syringomyelia is characterized by

(1) softening around the central canal of the cervical spinal cord
(2) loss of pain and temperature sense with segmental distribution
(3) sensory dissociation
(4) degeneration extending to the posterior funiculi

419. Subacute combined degeneration

(1) is associated with pernicious anemia
(2) usually affects the gray matter of the spinal cord
(3) causes posterior funiculi injury
(4) usually does not cause motor impairment

420. Alzheimer's disease is characterized by

(1) dementia
(2) neurofibrillary tangles
(3) diffuse general neuronal loss in the cortex, usually accentuated in the frontal and occipital lobes
(4) senile plaques

SUMMARY OF DIRECTIONS				
A	B	C	D	E
1, 2, 3 only	1, 3 only	2, 4 only	4 only	All are correct

421. Which of the following are NOT characteristic of glioblastoma multiforme?

(1) A uniform histologic pattern or grade
(2) A good prognosis
(3) Tumor cells with perinuclear "halos"
(4) Necrosis

DIRECTIONS: The groups of questions in this section consist of five lettered headings followed by several numbered items. For each numbered item choose the **one** lettered heading with which it is **most** closely associated. Each lettered heading may be used once, more than once, or not at all.

Questions 422-426
For each lesion, choose the lettered region in the diagram of the brain below in which it is most likely to occur.

422. Medulloblastoma

423. Hemangioblastoma

424. Chromophobe adenoma

425. Glioblastoma multiforme

426. Meningioma

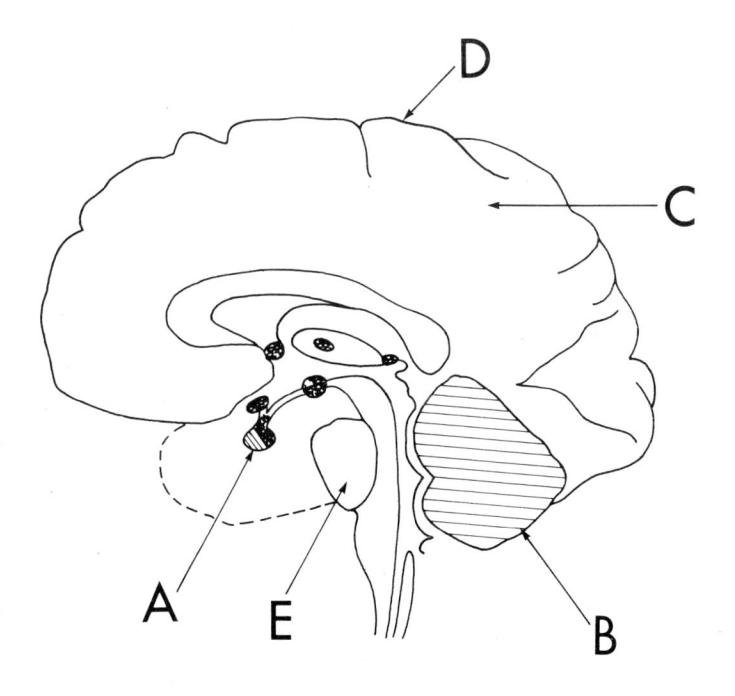

Questions 427-433
For each of the following diseases, choose the sign with which it is most likely to be associated.

(A) Cowdry A intranuclear inclusion body
(B) Disseminated focal demyelination
(C) Diffuse general demyelination
(D) Motor neuron disease
(E) Status spongiosus

427. Creutzfeldt-Jakob disease

428. Kuru

429. Subacute sclerosing panencephalitis

430. Krabbe's disease

431. Multiple sclerosis

432. Amyotrophic lateral sclerosis

433. Metachromatic leukodystrophy

Questions 434-439
For each disease, choose the sign with which it is most likely to be associated.

(A) Neurofibrillary tangles
(B) Lewy bodies
(C) Cowdry A intranuclear inclusion bodies
(D) Corpora amylacea
(E) None of the above

434. Idiopathic parkinsonism

435. Postencephalitic parkinsonism

436. Herpes simplex encephalitis

437. Alzheimer's disease

438. Cruetzfeldt-Jakob disease

439. Nonspecific postmortem finding not linked to a known disease process

Skeletomuscular System

DIRECTIONS: Each question below contains five suggested answers. Choose the **one best** response to each question.

440. The most common tumor that involves bone is

(A) a metastatic tumor from an extraosseous site
(B) osteogenic sarcoma
(C) multiple myeloma
(D) chondrosarcoma
(E) a giant cell tumor

441 Pott's disease (tuberculosis of the spine) most commonly involves

(A) cervical vertebrae
(B) cervical and thoracic vertebrae
(C) thoracic and lumbar vertebrae
(D) the sacroiliac region
(E) all regions of the vertebral column equally

442. The part of a long bone initially involved in hematogenous osteomyelitis is the

(A) metaphyseal region
(B) diaphysis
(C) epiphysis
(D) area around the entrance of the nutrient artery
(E) medullary cavity

443. Which of the following diseases is NOT a type of osteochondrosis?

(A) Osgood-Schlatter disease
(B) Legg-Calvé-Perthes disease
(C) Letterer-Siwe disease
(D) Freiberg's disease
(E) Osteochondritis dissecans

444. Arthritic involvement of only the distal interphalangeal joints is characteristic of

(A) rheumatoid arthritis
(B) Still's disease
(C) ankylosing spondylitis
(D) Reiter's disease
(E) psoriatic arthritis

445. The earliest radiologic sign of rheumatoid arthritis is

(A) soft tissue swelling
(B) soft tissue calcifications
(C) erosion of metacarpal heads
(D) "pen and egg-cup" deformity
(E) joint space narrowing

446. The lesion illustrated below is most likely to be

(A) a rheumatoid nodule
(B) myositis ossificans
(C) necrotizing panniculitis
(D) polymyositis
(E) fat necrosis

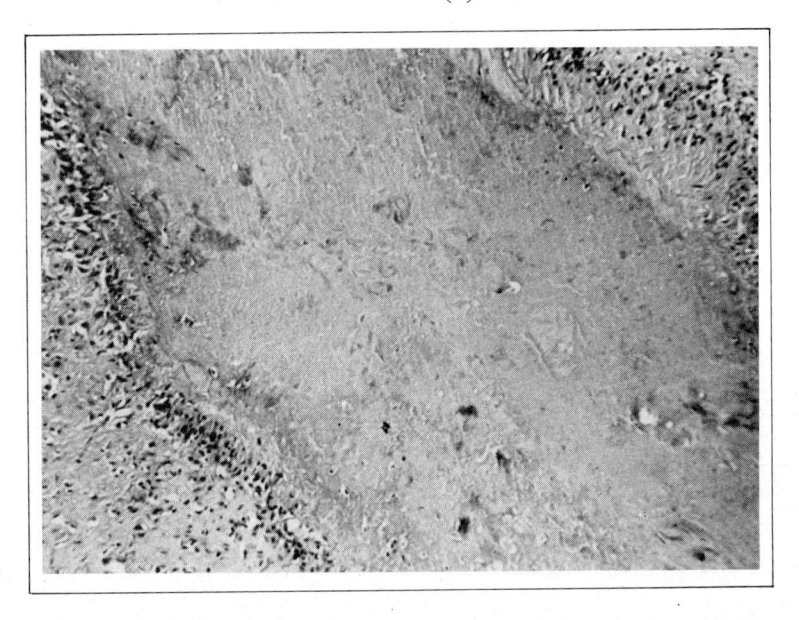

447. Bone metastases are most commonly associated with carcinoma of the

(A) kidney
(B) prostate
(C) pancreas
(D) intestine
(E) stomach

448. Osteomalacia has been shown to be the result of

(A) osteosarcoma
(B) excess vitamin D
(C) excess parathormone
(D) vitamin D deficiency
(E) vitamin A deficiency

449. Osteogenesis imperfecta involves

(A) defective synthesis of organic bone matrix
(B) lack of calcium absorption from the GI tract
(C) bone marrow aplasia
(D) absence of osteoblasts
(E) osteoclastic hyperactivity

450. The radiologic appearance of Ewing's sarcoma has been described as

(A) "onion skin"
(B) "sun ray"
(C) "soap bubble"
(D) "signet ring"
(E) "double bubble"

451. A patient presents with enlargement of the skull and bowing of the tibias and femurs. Radiologically, the bones are enlarged and have increased radiolucency. Based on this history and the bone biopsy shown below, the most likely diagnosis is

(A) osteomalacia
(B) osteoporosis
(C) Paget's disease
(D) dyschondroplasia
(E) osteogenesis imperfecta

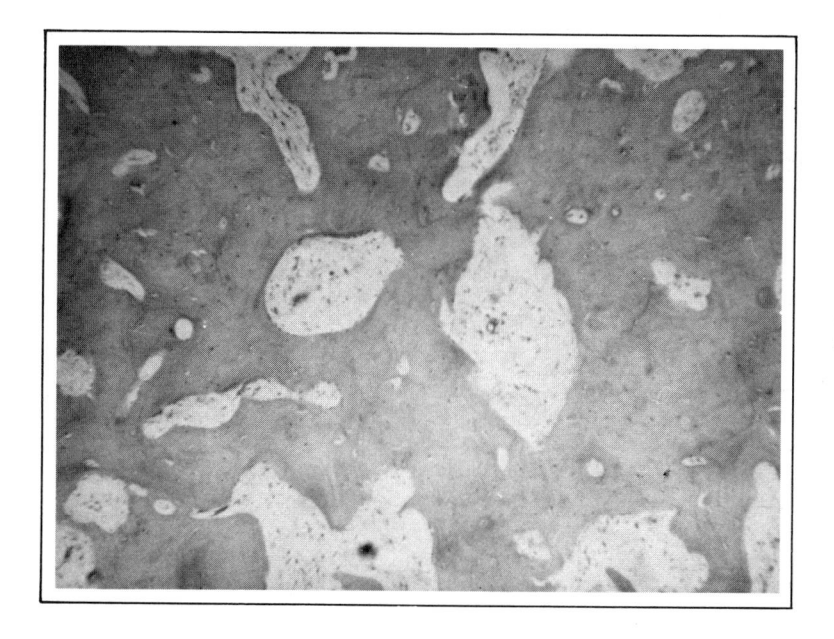

452. In comparison to the general population, workers using radium-containing paints have a higher incidence of

(A) osteogenic sarcoma
(B) carcinoma of the bladder
(C) carcinoma of the lung
(D) carcinoma of the skin
(E) leukemia

453. Which of the following disorders has an X-linked recessive pattern of transmission?

(A) Childhood muscular dystrophy
(B) Congenital adrenal hyperplasia
(C) Sphingomyelin lipidosis
(D) Renal tubular acidosis
(E) Hereditary spherocytosis

454. Malignant rhabdomyoblasts (elongated strap-shaped cells with cross-striations, or racket-shaped cells with eosinophilic cytoplasm), as pictured below, may be seen in all of the following lesions EXCEPT

(A) sarcoma botryoides
(B) myositis ossificans
(C) mixed heterologous müllerian tumor of uterus
(D) adult pleomorphic rhabdomyosarcoma
(E) embryonal rhabdomyosarcoma

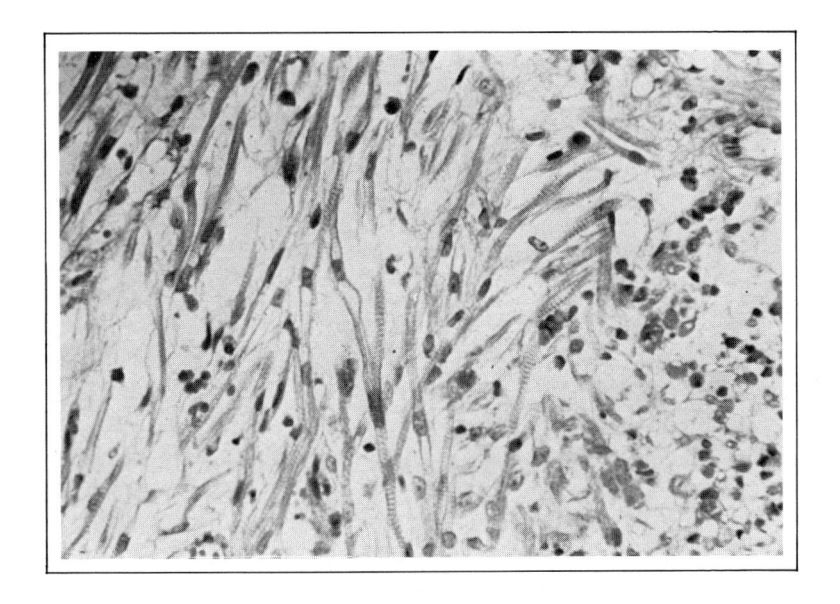

100

455. A perivascular inflammatory infiltrate in skeletal muscle as shown below, is likely to be seen in all of the following EXCEPT

(A) hypersensitivity angiitis
(B) polymyositis
(C) polyarteritis nodosa
(D) cystic medial necrosis
(E) systemic sclerosis

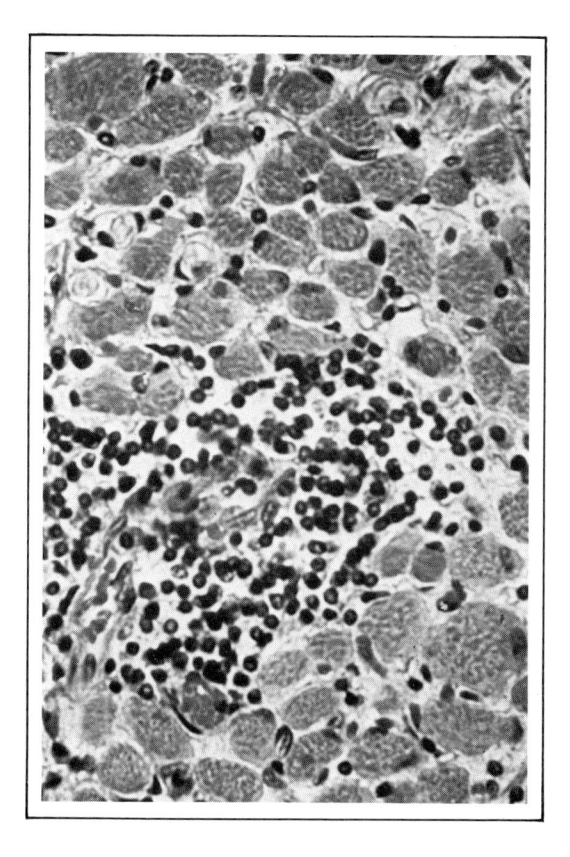

456. The thymus is thought to play a role in the pathogenesis of

(A) rheumatic fever
(B) myasthenia gravis
(C) giant cell arteritis
(D) diabetic glomerulosclerosis
(E) none of the above

DIRECTIONS: Each question below contains four suggested answers of which **one** or **more** is correct. Choose the answer

A	if	1, 2, and 3	are	correct
B	if	1 and 3	are	correct
C	if	2 and 4	are	correct
D	if	4	is	correct
E	if	1, 2, 3, and 4	are	correct

457. Juxtacortical (parosteal) osteosarcoma, shown below arising in the distal tibia,

(1) may be confused with myositis ossificans
(2) is primarily composed of cartilage
(3) has a much better prognosis than osteosarcoma arising within the bone shaft
(4) is usually secondary to trauma

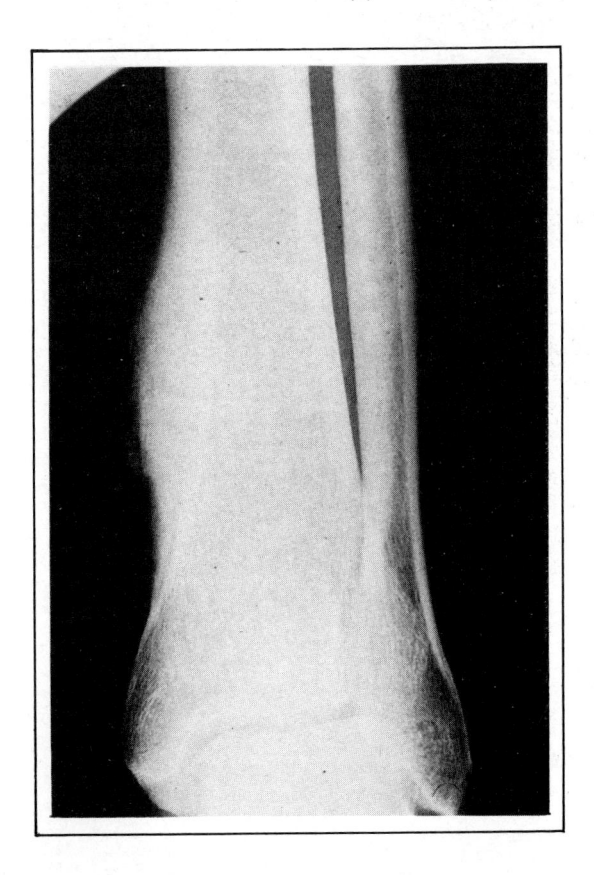

458. Osteogenic sarcoma, shown below in an x-ray of a hemisected tibia,

(1) is the most common type of bone cancer in the young
(2) may be associated with Paget's disease in the elderly
(3) may have a sun-burst apppearance on x-ray
(4) has a five-year survival of 50 percent

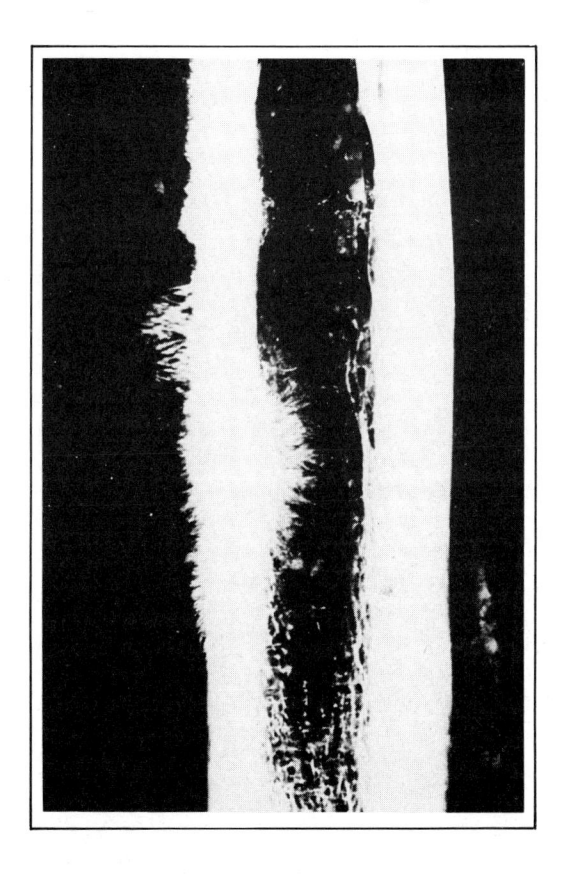

459. Bilateral calcifications of the menisci or cartilages of the knees is seen in

(1) hyperparathyroidism
(2) ochronosis
(3) gout
(4) chondrocalcinosis

SUMMARY OF DIRECTIONS

A	B	C	D	E
1, 2, 3 only	1, 3 only	2, 4 only	4 only	All are correct

460. Multiple, focal, osteolytic lesions in the skull, as shown below, are usually associated with

(1) increased production of monoclonal immunoglobulin
(2) prostatic carcinoma
(3) proliferation of neoplastic plasma cells
(4) Ewing's tumor

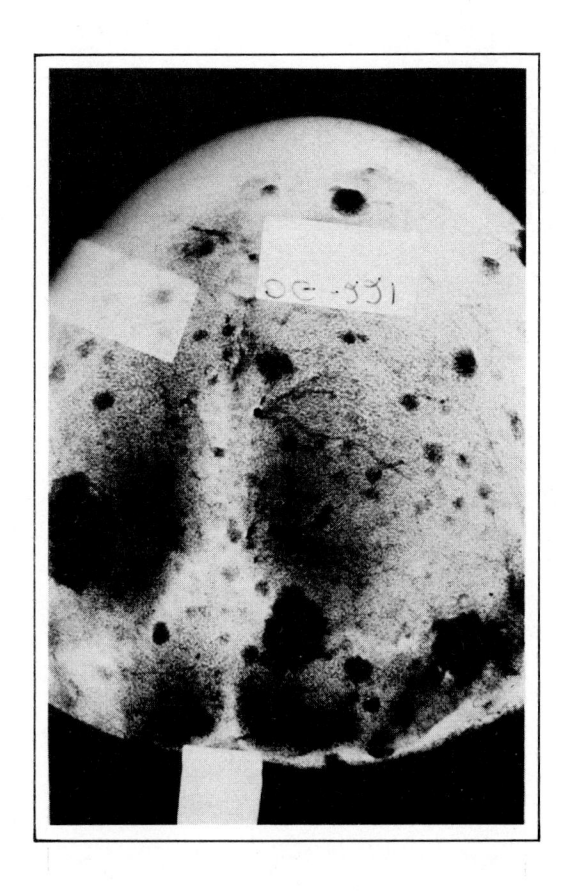

DIRECTIONS: The groups of questions in this section consist of five lettered headings followed by several numbered items. For each numbered item choose the **one** lettered heading with which it is **most** closely associated. Each lettered heading may be used once, more than once, or not at all.

Questions 461-465
For each bone lesion, select the lettered location and general configuration with which it is most likely to be associated in the diagram below.

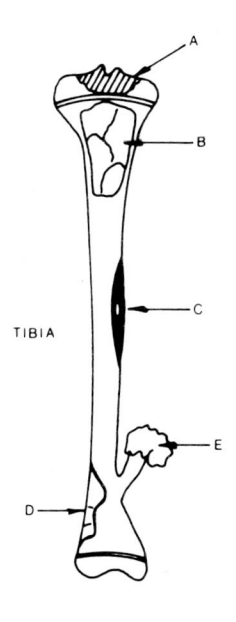

461. Giant cell tumor of bone (osteoclastoma)

462. Unicameral (solitary) bone cyst

463. Osteochondroma

464. Osteoid-osteoma

465. Non-ossifying fibroma of bone

Questions 466-470

For each disease, choose the artist's representation of a microradiogram, shown below, with which it is most likely to be associated. Answer "E" if the disease is not associated with any of the microradiograms.

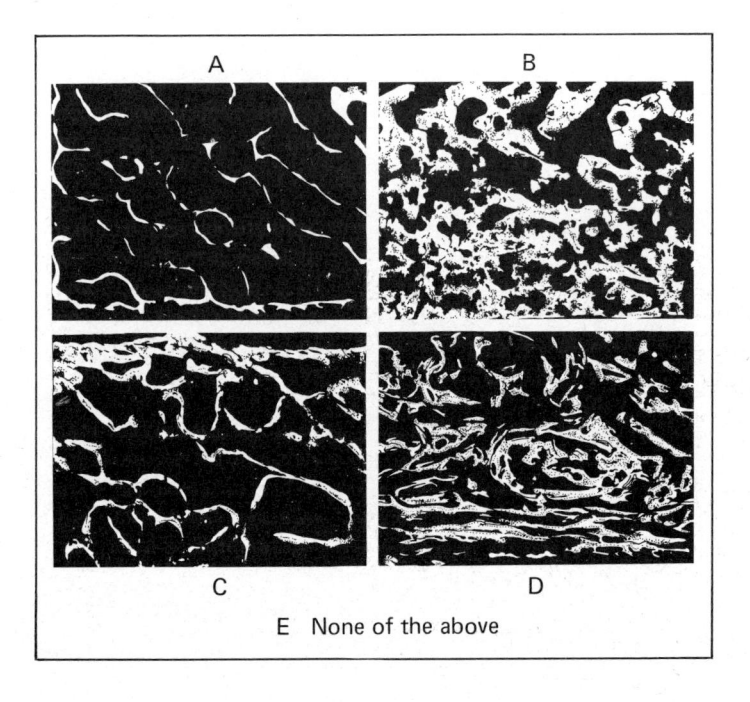

E None of the above

466. Osteosarcoma

467. Primary hyperparathyroidism

468. Vitamin D-resistant rickets

469. Osteoporosis

470. Paget's disease

Skin and Breast

DIRECTIONS: Each question below contains five suggested answers. Choose the **one best** response to each question.

471. The neoplasm illustrated below is the only human neoplasm which to date has been definitely shown to be caused by a virus. The lesion is a

(A) leukemic infiltrate
(B) renal cell carcinoma
(C) wart
(D) oat cell carcinoma
(E) basal cell carcinoma

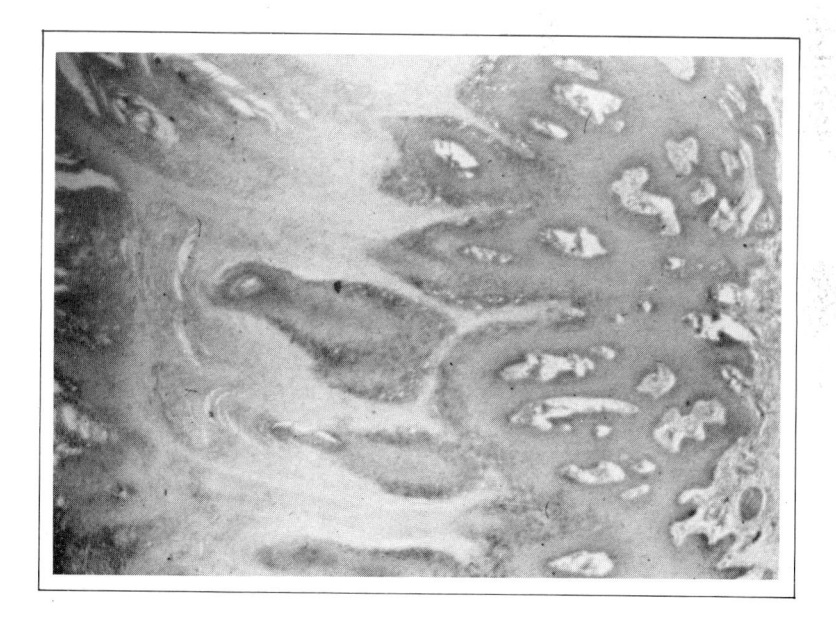

472. A brown, firm, localized facial skin lesion showing hyperkeratosis, acanthosis, an intact basal layer, and a normal dermis is most likely to be a

(A) malignant melanoma
(B) basal cell epithelioma
(C) verruca vulgaris
(D) solar keratosis
(E) seborrheic keratosis

473. The characteristic feature of urticaria pigmentosa is

(A) pustular rashes
(B) severe itching
(C) mast cell accumulation in the epidermis
(D) carotene-like pigmentation
(E) increased melanin pigmentation

474. In women between the age of 35 and 50 years, the most common cause of breast masses is

(A) carcinoma
(B) fibroadenoma
(C) fat necrosis
(D) cystic hyperplasia
(E) papilloma

475. Which of the following statements is NOT true?

(A) Women with cystic disease of the breast have a greater risk of developing breast carcinoma
(B) Cystic disease tends to be painful prior to the menstrual period
(C) Frequently, cystic disease regresses during pregnancy
(D) Cystic disease is rarely bilateral
(E) Cystic disease usually occurs in women at or near the menopause

476. Which of the following forms of breast cancer does NOT belong in the same classification as the others?

(A) Scirrhous carcinoma
(B) Lobular carcinoma
(C) Colloid or mucinous carcinoma
(D) Medullary carcinoma
(E) Ductal carcinoma

477. Which of the following forms of breast cancer has the most favorable prognosis?

(A) Infiltrating ductal carcinoma
(B) Scirrhous carcinoma
(C) Medullary carcinoma
(D) Colloid or mucinous carcinoma
(E) Cystosarcoma phyllodes

Questions 478-479

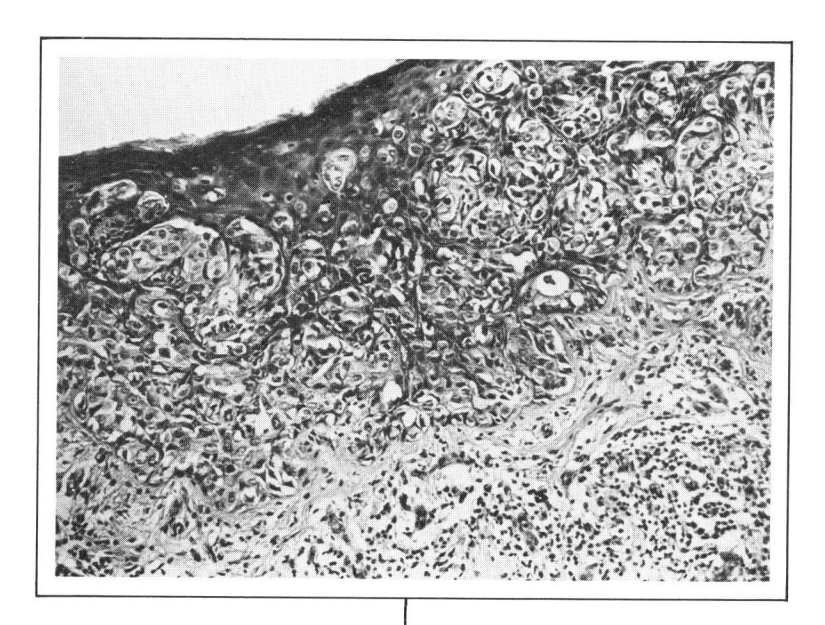

478. The lesion shown above was excised from the nipple of the left breast of a 42-year-old woman who complained of bloody discharge from the nipple for two months. The diagnosis is most likely to be

(A) epidermoid carcinoma
(B) acanthosis nigricans
(C) verruca vulgaris
(D) chronic inflammation
(E) Paget's disease of the nipple

479. The superficial nipple lesion shown above is almost invariably associated with

(A) gastrointestinal malignancy
(B) ductal adenocarcinoma of the breast
(C) multiple basal cell carcinomas
(D) collagen disease
(E) melanin production

480. The patient whose skin biopsy is illustrated below probably also has

(A) immune complex glomerulonephritis
(B) hilar lymphadenopathy
(C) discoid lupus
(D) infectious mononucleosis
(E) bacterial endocarditis

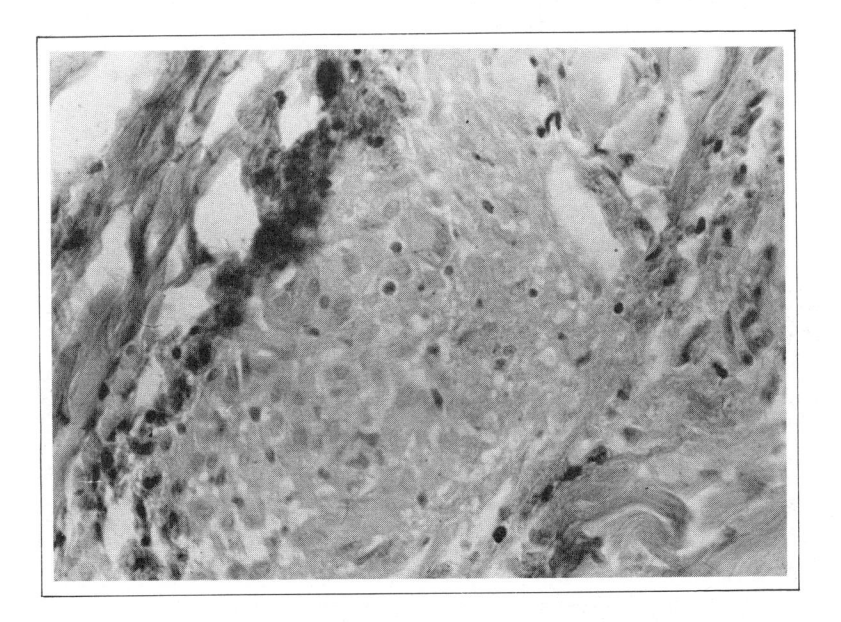

481. The pigmented skin lesion shown on the facing page should be

(A) excised and examined histologically
(B) fulgurated
(C) treated with topical 5-fluorouracil
(D) observed carefully
(E) treated with high dose x-ray

482. The subcutaneous nodule shown on the facing page was found on the scalp of a 9-year-old boy who had lived in Guatemala. The most likely diagnosis is

(A) onchocerciasis
(B) dracunculiasis
(C) loiasis
(D) filariasis
(E) ancylostomiasis

Photograph accompanies Question 481

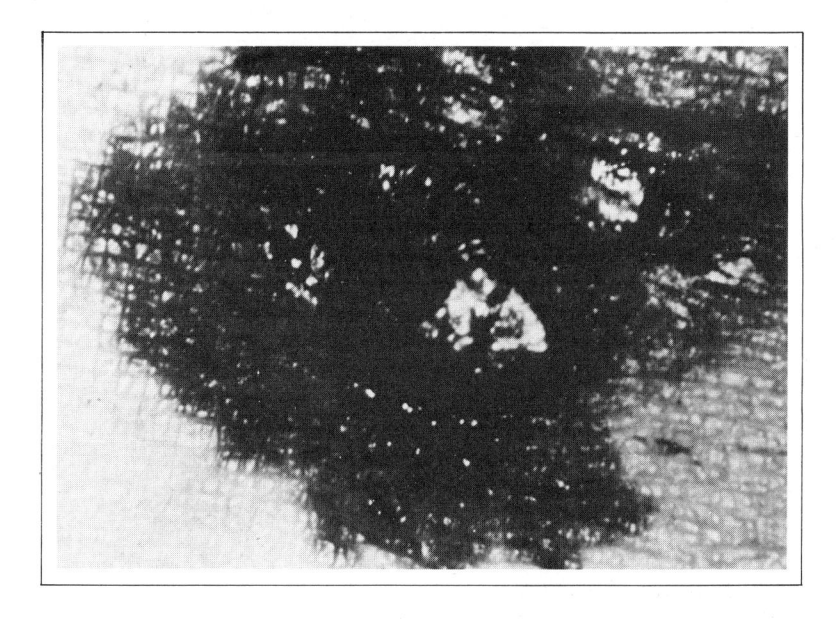

Photograph accompanies Question 482

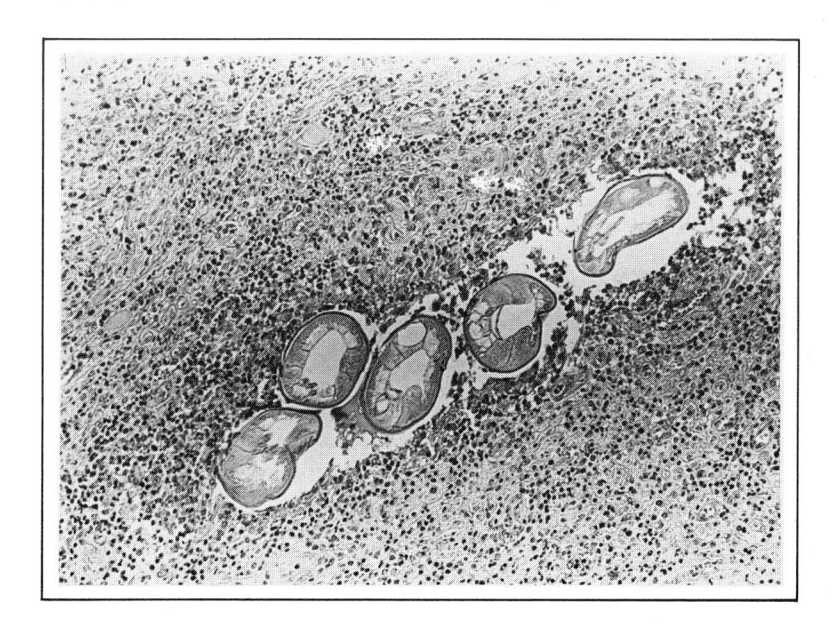

483. The fibrous tissue component of the common scirrhous carcinoma of the breast

(A) may metastasize
(B) may cause an extremely firm mass
(C) represents a coexistent fibrosarcoma
(D) is diagnostic of Paget's disease
(E) is a hamartoma

484. Most breast cancers arise from

(A) interductal stromal tissue
(B) ductal epithelium
(C) pre-existing adenomas
(D) traumatized breast tissue
(E) metaplastic fibrocytes

485. Cystic mammary dysplasia (fibrocystic disease)

(A) frequently leads to cancer
(B) should be treated by prophylactic simple mastectomy
(C) probably results from an exaggeration of the cyclic breast changes occurring during the menstrual cycle
(D) often occurs prior to puberty
(E) is usually iatrogenic

486. Enlargement of the breasts in a newborn infant may be caused by

(A) adrenal hyperplasia
(B) sarcoma botryoides
(C) supernumerary nipples
(D) delivery trauma
(E) maternal hormones

487. All of the following are congenital lesions EXCEPT

(A) mongolian spots
(B) ichthyosis
(C) port-wine stain (nevus flammeus)
(D) keratoacanthoma
(E) nevus vasculosus (strawberry hemangioma)

488. Acanthosis is common to all of the following skin lesions EXCEPT

(A) molluscum contagiosum
(B) psoriasis
(C) verruca vulgaris
(D) condyloma acuminatum
(E) scleroderma

DIRECTIONS: Each question below contains four suggested answers of which **one** or **more** is correct. Choose the answer

A	if	1, 2, and 3	are correct
B	if	1 and 3	are correct
C	if	2 and 4	are correct
D	if	4	is correct
E	if	1, 2, 3, and 4	are correct

489. Classic symptoms of hemochromatosis include

(1) skin pigmentation
(2) cirrhosis of the liver
(3) diabetes mellitus
(4) weight gain

490. Which of the following blistering skin lesions may be characterized by an intraepithelial location and intranuclear inclusion bodies?

(1) Varicella
(2) Variola
(3) Herpes simplex
(4) Erythema nodosum

491. Which of the following are considered to be premalignant lesions?

(1) Seborrheic keratosis
(2) Solar keratosis
(3) Fibroepithelial papilloma
(4) Leukoplakia

492. Melanin is present in

(1) the basal layer of the epidermis
(2) anthracotic nodules
(3) pigmented nevi
(4) heart-failure cells

493. Which of the following are characteristic histologic features of psoriasis?

(1) Parakeratosis
(2) Acanthosis
(3) Elongation of the rete ridges and dermal papillae
(4) Epidermal microabscesses containing polymorphonuclear neutrophilic leukocytes

494. Salivary gland tumors of low grade malignant potential include

(1) squamous cell carcinoma
(2) adenolymphoma (Warthin's tumor)
(3) undifferentiated carcinoma
(4) acinic cell tumor

SUMMARY OF DIRECTIONS

A	B	C	D	E
1, 2, 3 only	1, 3 only	2, 4 only	4 only	All are correct

495. Breast cancer is more common in a woman

    (1) with an early menarche
    (2) with previous breast disease
    (3) with a family history of breast cancer
    (4) who is multiparous

496. Which of the following usually do NOT give rise to palpable breast masses?

    (1) Gross cystic disease
    (2) Solitary intraductal papilloma
    (3) Traumatic fat necrosis
    (4) Lobular carcinoma in situ

DIRECTIONS: The group of questions in this section consists of five lettered headings followed by several numbered items. For each numbered item choose the **one** lettered heading with which it is **most** closely associated. Each lettered heading may be used once, more than once, or not at all.

Questions 497-500
For each of the following descriptions, choose the skin lesion with which it is associated.

(A) Acanthosis nigricans
(B) Juvenile melanoma
(C) Malignant melanoma
(D) Blue nevus
(E) Halo nevus

497. Characterized by clinical depigmentation of the skin and chronic inflammation of the dermis

498. A form of compound nevus that often shows histologic atypia with giant cells, and is erroneously diagnosed as malignant

499. A papillomatous, pigmented lesion of the skin associated with visceral malignancy in adults over 40 years old

500. Elevated, dark-colored lesion structurally related to the mongolian spot or nevus of Ota

General Pathology

1. **The answer is C.** *(Robbins, 1974. p 13.)* An organ or tissue may enlarge in response to a variety of stimuli. Enlargement may be due to an increase in the size of individual cells (hypertrophy), or an increase in cell number (hyperplasia). Cellular hypertrophy consists of the production of more cellular organelles, such as mitochondria or endoplasmic reticulum.

2. **The answer is B.** *(Robbins, 1974. p 13.)* Hypertrophy refers to an increase in cell size which causes an increase in the size of an organ without an increase in cell number. Cardiac and skeletal muscles respond to an increased work load by hypertrophy, rather than by hyperplasia.

3. **The answer is C.** *(Robbins, 1974. p 89.)* The cells of the body can be divided into three groups based on their regenerative ability. Labile cells continue to proliferate throughout life. Stable cells can proliferate if necessary but do not normally do so. Permanent cells cannot reproduce themselves. Regeneration is limited to cells of the first two categories and connective tissue is composed of both.

4. **The answer is B.** *(Robbins, 1974. p 71.)* Polymorphonuclear leukocytes are usually the first cells to appear in a focus of acute inflammation. Their major roles include phagocytosis, release of lytic lysosomal enzymes, and the formation of chemotactic factors. The trimolecular complex of complement (C5, 6, and 7) is activated by neutrophil esterases to yield an attractant for neutrophils. Mononuclear cells are also attracted to neutrophil products.

5. **The answer is A.** *(Robbins, 1974. p 17.)* Metaplasia may represent an adaptive substitution, for cells that are sensitive to environmental stress, of other cell types better able to withstand adverse conditions. For example, in chronic respiratory irritation secondary to cigarette smoking, the normal columnar ciliated epithelial cells of the trachea and bronchi are often replaced by stratified squamous epithelial cells (squamous metaplasia).

6. **The answer is D.** *(Anderson, ed 6. pp 40-42.)* Lymphocytes are most often associated with chronic inflammation and delayed immune reactions although the other cells listed can participate.

7. **The answer is B.** *(Anderson, ed 6. p 46.)* Catarrhal inflammation involves mucous membranes and superficial tissues and results in copious secretion of mucus.

8. **The answer is D.** *(Robbins, 1974. p 350.)* The kidney is often the organ most severely damaged by shock. It becomes pale and the pyramids become cyanotic and congested. Microscopically the cells of the distal convoluted tubules can be seen to be swollen or dead. These changes are called acute tubular necrosis.

9. **The answer is C.** *(Takahashi, 1971. pp 203-205.)* Marked variation in cell size, nuclear hyperchromatism, and prominent nuclear membranes are diagnostic for malignancy. The tendency of cells to cluster and overlap, the prominent nucleoli, and the vacuolated cytoplasm strongly suggest adenocarcinoma rather than oat cell carcinoma.

10. **The answer is A.** *(Robbins, 1974. p 540.)* In general, cells are sensitive to irradiation in direct proportion to their mitotic activity and in inverse proportion to their level of specialization. Lymphocytes and their tumors (lymphomas), are the notable exceptions to this generalization. The radiosensitivity of a tumor often parallels the sensitivity of its cell of origin, as is the case in the highly radiosensitive germ cells of the testes and the seminoma.

11. **The answer is B.** *(Robbins, 1974. p 889.)* Ninety percent of oral cavity malignancies are squamous cell carcinomas of which half arise in the tongue. The prognosis depends on the degree of cellular differentiation, the extent of spread, and the presence of lymph node metastases. Generally, metastases are confined to nodes above the clavicles, but lung, liver, and bone may be involved later in the disease.

12. **The answer is D.** *(Davidsohn, ed 15. p 1261.)* In a patient with suspected meningitis, microscopic examination of cerebrospinal fluid is of immediate importance. In the photograph shown, all the cells are polymorphonuclear leukocytes and bacteria are visible in the cytoplasm. Neutrophils may be present in viral or tuberculous meningitis, but lymphocytes are more common. Demonstration of bacteria by Gram stain of the CSF is the crucial test, and in early bacterial meningitis it will be positive in greater than 90 percent of cases.

13. **The answer is C.** *(Robbins, 1974. p 121.)* Carcinomas tend to spread via the lymphatic system, while sarcomas preferentially embolize through blood vessels. (These generalizations are not, however, absolutes.) Regional lymph nodes are frequently excised at the time of removal of the primary tumor in the case of a carcinoma, but not a sarcoma. Hematogenous tumor emboli most frequently involve the liver and lungs.

14. **The answer is D.** *(Robbins, 1974. pp 124-125.)* The number of metastases lodging in a given organ is largely a function of the richness of its blood supply and its volume of blood flow. Notable exceptions are skeletal muscles and the spleen.

15. **The answer is A.** *(Davidshohn, ed 15. p 1052.)* Enterobius vermicularis (pinworm) is a common parasitic nematode. The eggs are rarely found in stool specimens, so the tape swab is essential to identify the organism. The eggs have a thick, hyaline shell, often with a flattened side, and usually contain a curled larva. The eggs measure approximately 25 by 50 µ. The other parasites listed are best identified from stool specimens and have a different appearance.

16. **The answer is B.** *(Anderson, ed 8. p 311.)* Extension by the lymphatics is the common method of spread of carcinoma. Tumor cells grow into lymphatic channels and are broken off and carried as emboli to draining lymph nodes. The tumor is lodged initially in the subcapsular space or peripheral sinus. The tumor then grows within the lymph node and eventually spreads throughout the node and onward in the lymphatic system.

17. **The answer is D.** *(Robbins, 1974. p 156.)* Interlacing bundles of anaplastic spindle cells characterize fibrosarcoma. The extreme variations in nuclear size and shape, and the presence of bizarre giant cells help to differentiate this tumor from a benign fibroma.

18. **The answer is B.** *(Robbins, 1974. p 37.)* Alcoholic hyalin within ethanol-damaged hepatocytes ultrastructurally has been shown to be composed of closely packed fibrils, as seen in the illustration.

19. **The answer is A.** *(Robbins, 1974. p 300.)* Niemann-Pick disease is characterized by the accumulation of sphingomyelin in the reticuloendothelial cells of the liver, spleen, bone marrow, and lymph nodes. Most cases also involve the brain. In classic cases, patients have a deficiency of the sphingomyelin-cleaving enzyme sphingomyelinase. The diagnosis can be confirmed by demonstration of vacuolation and degeneration of ganglion cells in biopsies of the rectal wall.

20. **The answer is B.** *(Robbins, 1974. p 305.)* The Hand-Schüller-Christian complex or histiocytosis X consists of three syndromes: Letterer-Siwe disease; Hand-Schüller-Christian syndrome; and eosinophilic granuloma. All consist of abnormal proliferation of histiocytes containing varying amounts of lipids.

21. **The answer is A.** *(Beeson, ed 13. p 1809.)* Pathologic changes seen commonly in patients with Klinefelter's syndrome include atrophy and hyalinization of the seminiferous tubules. The atrophy gives rise to small testes which are usually firmer than normal and the azoospermia is a result of the seminiferous tubule dysgensis. Urinary gonadotropins are elevated in primary hypogonadism in contrast to that secondary to pituitary disease. Gynecomastia is caused by androgen deficiency.

22. The answer is A. *(Beeson, ed 13. p 1717.)* Laurence-Moon-Biedl syndrome is characterized by mental retardation, retinitis pigmentosa, hypogonadism, adiposity, and polydactyly. A number of cases have been associated with sex chromosome aneuploidy.

23. The answer is A. *(Anderson, ed 6. pp 322-323.)* The features described are characteristic of chronic granulomatous disease and involve the inability of leukocytes to destroy certain phagocytized bacteria.

24. The answer is D. *(Robbins, 1974. p 500.)* Nicotinamide (niacinamide) is a functional component of two important coenzymes involved in electron transport. Deficiency may develop as a result of severe malnourishment or in disease states such as chronic alcoholism. Nicotinamide deficiency leads to pellagra, a disease characterized by dermatitis, diarrhea, and dementia.

25. The answer is A. *(Robbins, 1974. pp 246, 1065.)* Diseases of the salivary glands such as mumps, Mikulicz syndrome, or inflammation of the pancreas, may cause elevations of the serum amylase. Elevated amylase may also be produced by other conditions affecting the upper abdomen such as a perforated duodenal ulcer impinging on the pancreas.

26. The answer is E. *(Robbins, 1974, p 519.)* Methanol exerts its prime toxic effect after its oxidation to formaldehyde and formic acid. These substances cause degeneration of the receptor cells of the retina. Swelling of the brain and brain stem may also occur.

27. The answer is A. *(Robbins, 1974. pp 37-38.)* Fibrinoid is an eosinophilic, amorphous material that contains various plasma proteins, most importantly the immunoglobulins and complement. Fibrinoid usually appears in the foci of immunologic injury, as in the Arthus reaction.

28. The answer is E. *(Stanbury, ed 3. p 1033.)* In Wilson's disease (hepatolenticular degeneration), increased copper is localized in the cornea giving rise to the characteristic Kayser-Fleischer corneal rings. Other clinical features of the disease include pseudosclerosis, cirrhosis, and hypersplenism. The basic abnormality in Wilson's disease has not yet been elucidated.

29. The answer is A. *(Anderson, ed 6. pp 87-88.)* Homogentisic acid localizes in the cartilage and is associated with alkaptonuria. The genetic defect in alkaptonuria results in the absence of the enzyme homogentisic acid oxidase. Homogentisic acid produced during the metabolism of phenylalanine and tyrosine therefore accumulates and may be excreted in the urine. The pigment deposited in ochronosis is presumably a polymer derivative of homogentisic acid but its exact chemical structure has not yet been determined.

30. The answer is D. *(Anderson, ed 6. pp 84-85.)* Gout probably results from an enzymatic defect in purine catabolism and from faulty renal tubular excretion of uric acid. The disease manifests itself primarily in the joints and produces a characteristic form of acute and chronic arthritis presumably as a result of the presence of crystals of sodium urate. The cardinal feature of this disease is hyperuricemia. Primary gout reflects an inborn error of metabolism. In secondary gout the hyperuricemia is either a manifestation of an acquired disorder with rapid tissue turnover, or of the use of certain drugs.

31. The answer is C. *(Davidshohn, ed 15. p 296.)* When the serum of an individual with systemic lupus erythematosus (SLE) is incubated with a mixture of damaged and healthy neutrophils, some of the normal leukocytes will be found to contain a large, homogeneous, purple cytoplasmic mass. The purple mass is composed of nuclear material from the damaged neutrophils that has been altered by a serum antibody. In the absence of the SLE factor, nucleophagocytosis may also occur, but the structural integrity of the ingested nucleus will be retained (tart cells).

32. The answer is A. *(Anderson, ed 6. p 76.)* McArdle's disease and Pompe's disease while classified as glycogenoses do not result from a glucose 6-phosphatase deficiency in liver and kidney cells. McArdle's disease is characterized by a lack of muscle phosphorylase, high muscle glycogen concentrations, and normal muscle phosphorylase kinase activities. Pompe's disease reflects a deficiency in lysosomal α-glucosidase with accumulation of glycogen within lysosomes. The Crigler-Najjar and Gilbert syndromes are hereditary hyperbilirubinemias. Crigler-Najjar syndrome appears to be the result of severe icterus due to defective conjugation of bilirubin, while Gilbert syndrome is a low-grade, chronic, unconjugated hyperbilirubinemia with normal values for direct-reacting bilirubin.

33. The answer is C. *(Anderson, ed 6. p 505.)* An allograft is also called a homograft and refers to grafts between members of the same species. An autograft refers to a tissue graft taken from one site and placed in a different site in the same individual. Isografts are grafts between individuals from an inbred strain of animals. A graft between individuals of two different species is a xenograft or heterograft.

34. The answer is C. *(Robbins, 1974. pp 239-242.)* Fifteen to twenty percent of cases of polymyositis are associated with underlying visceral malignancies of virtually any organ. Although the cause of this association remains unknown, it has been postulated that some cancers either produce products that are toxic to skeletal muscle, or that the tumors contain antigens cross-reactive with skeletal muscle.

35. **The answer is B.** *(Robbins, 1974. p 236.)* Lupus erythematosus is a multisystem disease, but the most ominous prognostic sign is the development of nephritis. In addition to renal failure, causes of death include cardiac failure, central nervous system disease, hemorrhage, and bacterial infections which are probably related to the immunosuppressive therapy used to control the primary disease.

36. **The answer is B.** *(Davidsohn, ed 15. pp 301, 1235.)* Antinuclear antibodies are found in a number of diseases. Several different types are found in patients with systemic lupus, and it is in this disease that the highest titers are found. The antinuclear antibodies of periarteritis, malignancies, and chronic active hepatitis are less commonly found and are usually seen in very low titers. In poststreptococcal glomerulonephritis, antigen-antibody complexes deposited at basement membranes are the characteristic finding.

37. **The answer is C.** *(Stanbury, ed 3. p 513.)* Familial high-density lipoprotein deficiency, Tangier disease, is characterized by almost complete absence of high-density lipoprotein and by storage of cholesterol esters in body tissues. The low plasma cholesterol concentration with normal or elevated triglycerides and the distinctive yellow-orange coloration of affected tissues are said to be pathognomic for this disease.

38. **The answer is D.** *(Stanbury, ed 3. p 992.)* Xanthinuria is a result of a gross deficiency of xanthine oxidase, which is responsible for the conversion of xanthine to uric acid. Xanthine, therefore, replaces uric acid as a urinary end-product. Xanthinuria is a very rare autosomal recessive disorder, and less than a dozen well-documented cases have been reported.

39. **The answer is A.** *(Stanbury, ed 3. p 1295.)* Hypophosphatasia is a familial disease in which severe skeletal defects result from a failure of deposition of apatite in osteoid and of normal ossification at epiphyseal plates. Both plasma and urine contain excessive levels of phosphoryl ethanolamine. Other clinical findings may include hypercalcemia, renal damage, and premature synostosis of the cranial bones.

40. **The answer is A.** *(Davidsohn, ed 15. pp 1231-1232.)* While several antibodies may be present in the serum of a person with primary biliary cirrhosis, the presence of antimitochondrial antibodies is most specific. This antibody is seen in other forms of liver disease but much less commonly. Smooth muscle antibodies are sometimes seen in chronic active hepatitis, antinuclear antibodies in lupus, and Dane particles (antigenic structures) in acute type B viral hepatitis.

41. The answer is B. *(Davidshohn, ed 15. p 1233.)* Rheumatoid factor (RF) is an IgM with specificity for IgG. Rheumatoid factor is not present at all times in patients classified as having rheumatoid arthritis and is often lacking in some of the rheumatoid variants. Other inflammatory disease states may be associated with the presence of rheumatoid factor; joint involvement is not required. RF is not an antisynovial antibody.

42. The answer is A. *(Davidshohn, ed 15. p 1229.)* C-reactive protein (CRP) elevations, as well as elevations in the erythrocyte sedimentation rate (ESR) are nonspecific markers of inflammatory conditions. The CRP rises faster and returns to normal earlier than the ESR in most inflammatory diseases. Most bacterial illnesses, rheumatoid arthritis, rheumatic fever, and diseases leading to necrosis and tissue damage will elevate the CRP. Significant elevation of the CRP is usually not seen in viral illnesses.

43. The answer is C. *(Davidshohn, ed 15. pp 1220-1222.)* The RPR, Kolmer test, and VDRL are rapid, easy serologic tests that identify the presence of antibodies against treponemal or cardiolipin-lipid antigens. Biologic false positive reactions are not uncommon in these tests because of their somewhat low specificity; because they are easy to perform, the tests are still used for screening patients. The TPI and FTA-ABS are tests for treponemal antigen, and although technically more difficult have greater specificity. The FTA-ABS is generally the most sensitive and specific of the syphilis testing procedures.

44. The answer is A. *(Anderson, ed 6. pp 333-334.)* Tuberculoid leprosy results when intense host resistance to the infecting organism is present. The inflammatory reaction is destructive especially to nerves which are infiltrated and destroyed. The infiltrate usually extends to the epidermis. Large numbers of bacilli are *not* seen and are more characteristic of lepromatous leprosy.

45. The answer is D. *(Robbins, 1974. p 389.)* The causative microbe of granuloma inguinale is a pleomorphic coccobacillus, *Donovania granulomatis*. Tissue biopsies, or impression smears stained by the Wright method, usually reveal these microbes situated primarily within the monocytes, although a small number of extracellular microorganisms may be seen. The intracellular forms are referred to as Donovan bodies.

46. The answer is E. *(Anderson, ed 6. pp 356-362.)* Lymphogranuloma venereum is caused by an agent of the psittacosis group and has been variously classified by authors as bacterial, viral, and most recently chlamydial. The disease usually appears as a genital skin infection with rapid spread to regional lymph nodes. Occasionally, it can present as a systemic involvement with lesions present in the brain, meninges, lungs, kidneys, bones, and joints. The other infections mentioned are caused by nonvenereal spirochetes.

47. **The answer is E.** *(Davidsohn, ed 15. p 1263.)* Elevations in CSF globulins often occur in multiple sclerosis and other demyelinating diseases. An abnormal band on electrophoresis may occur even in the absence of elevated globulins. Late tertiary syphilis may exhibit these findings, but they would not be seen in the secondary stage. Tumor or meningeal leukemia can also produce elevated CSF globulin levels but the presence of tumor cells and absence of an electrophoretic band would lead to the proper diagnosis.

48. **The answer is A.** *(Davidsohn, ed 15. pp 1281-1282.)* While human chorionic gonadotropin (HCG) levels are characteristically elevated in all the conditions listed, up to 50 percent of patients with an ectopic pregnancy may have urine levels of HCG less than 1.0 IU/ml. Since many of the pregnancy tests used do not detect levels in this range, a negative test for urinary HCG does not rule out an ectopic pregnancy.

49. **The answer is D.** *(Davidsohn, ed 15. p 876.)* People with the genetic disease cystic fibrosis (mucoviscidosis) exhibit a variety of abnormalities of exocrine gland secretion. All exocrine glands are affected, but the sweat glands are most accessible for diagnostic testing. Secretions are increased in viscosity and concentration of sodium as well as chloride. The test is highly specific and sensitive if properly performed.

50. **The answer is B.** *(Davidsohn, ed 15. pp 625-627.)* The combination of a normal serum triglyceride and markedly elevated cholesterol level indicates type II lipoproteinemia. Type II individuals frequently have tendonous and corneal xanthomas, premature atherosclerosis, and a family history of lipid abnormalities. The other types of hyperlipoproteinemia generally produce an elevation in serum triglycerides. Type II is the only type in which visual examination generally reveals a clear serum.

51. **The answer is A.** *(Davidsohn, ed 15. pp 602, 607-609.)* Most healthy individuals exhibit a peak blood glucose level 30 to 45 minutes after ingestion of a 100 gram glucose load, with return to normal values after 90 to 120 minutes. In the figure shown: "B" represents "chemical diabetes;" "C" shows an abnormal response with a dip into low glucose; "D" may represent malabsorption; and "E" is an overtly diabetic curve.

52. **The answer is A.** *(Davidsohn, ed 15. p 849.)* The curve shown is that of SGOT. CPK rises and declines more rapidly. LDH declines much more slowly. Alkaline phosphatase and 5′-nucleotidase are not normally elevated after a myocardial infarct.

53. **The answer is D.** *(Davidshohn, ed 15. pp 642-644.)* Parathyroid hormone (PTH) acts to increase plasma calcium levels and decrease serum phosphate levels by its action on three main target organs: bone, kidney, and intestinal mucosa. Mobilization of calcium from bone is the major action and is accomplished by osteocytic and osteoclastic osteolysis. PTH enhances renal tubular reabsorption of calcium and decreases reabsorption of phosphate by its effect on renal tubular cells. The least sensitive target is the intestinal mucosa where PTH may promote absorption of dietary calcium.

54. **The answer is C.** *(Davidshohn, ed 15. pp 793-796.)* Vomiting leads to loss of hydrogen and chloride ions, resulting in a hypochloremic alkalosis. Liver disease is associated with either respiratory alkalosis or metabolic acidosis. Aspirin ingestion, diabetes, and shock lead to metabolic acidosis.

55. **The answer is B.** *(Anderson, ed 6. p 382.)* Encephalitis lethargica appeared during World War I and was endemic in many regions of the world through 1925. The neurologic sequelae of this epidemic encephalitis include parkinsonian states, dementias, spasticities, dystonias, and oculogyric crises. The consequences were seen in some patients immediately following recovery from the acute encephalitis, while in other individuals a latent period of ten years or more passed before the onset of the chronic sequelae. This fact led to speculation that either a continuing chronic infection by the encephalitic virus was the cause or that neuronal degeneration had occurred. Neither of these explanations has been proven.

56. **The answer is C.** *(Davidshohn, ed 15. pp 721-722.)* The urinary 17-ketogenic steroid determination measures 17-hydroxysteroids and additional metabolites. The measurement of urinary 17-ketosteroids gives information about androgen metabolites but not glucocorticoid activity. Plasma cortisol and aldosterone levels fluctuate widely and although useful for some purposes, do not reflect cumulative daily activity.

57. **The answer is A.** *(Davidshohn, ed 15. pp 870-873.)* Although an elevated serum amylase level is usually associated with pancreatitis, it can be associated with mumps (viral pancreatitis), renal disease (decreased clearance), ruptured ectopic pregnancy (multiple causes), and morphine administration (decreased excretion). Diabetes leads to hypoamylasemia which is a rare laboratory finding. The reason may be related to the correlation between amylase activity and albumin and calcium concentrations. Low values have also been reported in patients with serum protein loss in congestive heart failure, gastrointestinal cancer, fracture, pleurisy, and intestinal obstruction.

58. The answer is A. *(Davidshohn, ed 15. pp 86-88.)* Urinary clearance is equal to the concentration of a compound excreted per unit of time divided by the serum concentration of that compound:

$$\frac{(361 \text{ mg}/770\text{ml}) (770 \text{ ml}/1440 \text{ min})}{.02 \text{ mg}/100 \text{ ml}} = 12.5 \text{ ml/min}.$$

59. The answer is B. *(Davidshohn, ed 15. pp 44, 597.)* Consumption of a large amount of cranberry juice will acidify urine and promote formation of uric acid calculi from uric acid which is relatively insoluble at low pHs. An alkaline urine would be preferred in a patient with severe hyperuricemia since the uric acid would then remain in solution. Acid urine may also be produced by a diet high in meat protein, but citrus fruits, paradoxically, will produce alkaline urine.

60. The answer is B. *(Davidshohn, ed 15. pp 588-589.)* Bence Jones protein and light chain protein are synonymous. Bence Jones proteins are found in the urine of approximately 50 percent of people with multiple myeloma and represent heat-precipitable immunoglobulin light chains (kappa or lambda). The M-component in multiple myeloma is usually IgG, IgA, or Bence Jones, and rarely IgD.

61. The answer is E. *(Davidshohn, ed 15. p 571.)* Routine serum immunoelectrophoresis is performed using clotted blood. Since fibrinogen is consumed in the process of clotting, it does not appear in the electrophoretic scan. When the electrophoresis is done on plasma, or partially clotted whole blood, the fibrinogen peak will appear between the beta and gamma globulin regions.

62. The answer is D. *(Davidshohn, ed 15. pp 847-848.)* Erythrocytes and platelets, as well as prostatic tissue contain a phosphatase which is active at acid pH values. The phosphatase may be released in polycythemia or prostatic diseases. In the other diseases listed, the serum level of this enzyme is usually normal.

63. The answer is A. *(Davidshohn, ed 15. p 751.)* The hyperthyroidism of Graves' disease is associated with an elevated level of LATS. The level of TSH is usually low in Graves' disease. The other hormones listed are not associated with the pituitary-thyroid axis and their levels are not appreciably altered.

64. The answer is A. *(Robbins, 1974. p 442.)* Fungi can be identified in tissue sections by their affinity for silver stains. Fungal infections are uncommon except in those patients who are particularly vulnerable because of debilitation due to malignancy or immunosuppression by drugs or irradiation. Many fungal infections are confined to the skin, but almost any organ can be involved in a susceptible host.

65. The answer is A. *(Davidshohn, ed 15. pp 854-855.)* The patient described probably has hepatitis. Liver cells contain higher proportions of LDH$_4$ and LDH$_5$ than do myocardium or red blood cells, both of which contain greater relative amounts of LDH$_1$ and LDH$_2$. Lung is high in LDH$_3$ and brain tissue contains only small amounts of LDH$_5$.

66. The answer is C. *(Robbins, 1974. p 449.)* The main distinguishing feature of the Mucorales, histologically, is the lack of septa in their hyphae. Mucorales are fungi of low virulence, and are opportunistic invaders in chronically debilitated patients, especially immunosuppressed patients and individuals with advanced diabetes mellitus. PAS stains the fungi, and is particularly useful in demonstrating the large, branching, hyphae.

67. The answer is D. *(Davidshohn, ed 15. pp 742-743.)* T$_3$ is the thyroid hormone with the greatest physiologic activity, although T$_4$ is present in greater quantities and thus is usually the best measure of thyroid activity. MIT and DIT are not released from the gland and have little activity. Thyroglobulin is the carrier protein for binding stored thyroid hormones.

68. The answer is E. *(Stanbury, ed 3. p 1065.)* Since excessive absorption of iron requires several decades to accumulate, 80 percent of patients with primary hemochromatosis become symptomatic only after the age of 40. Patients with this disease may accumulate 20 to 60 grams of iron in their tissues during a 50-year period.

69. The answer is D. *(Stanbury, ed 3. p 889.)* Hyperuricemia is the main biochemical feature of primary gout. Asymptomatic hyperuricemia is the early stage of primary gout during which the serum urate level is raised but arthritic symptoms are not yet apparent. In certain individuals the disease progresses to recurrent attacks of acute gouty arthritis and/or renal lithiasis.

70. The answer is C. *(Stanbury, ed 3. p 857.)* The adrenogenital syndrome associated with adrenocortical hyperplasia is a genetic disorder in the biosynthesis of adrenal corticoids. Certain forms of the syndrome result in renal excretion of sodium leading to severe salt-wasting and addisonian-like crises. The "salt-losing" form of the disease has been reported to occur in between 30 and 65 percent of all cases of the genetic disorder.

71. The answer is B. *(Stanbury, ed 3. p 615.)* Tay-Sachs disease is a biochemical abnormality of the nervous system in which ganglion cells and proliferating glial cells contain large amounts of gangliosides. Over 90 percent of the accumulated gangliosides are monosialogangliosides lacking the terminal galactose found in most gangliosides in normal brain. The excessive accumulation of this material is accompanied by myelin degeneration.

72. The answer is E. *(Stanbury, ed 3. p 127.)* Pentosuria represents an inborn error of metabolism for which no functional disturbance has been demonstrated. It results in the excretion of 1 to 4 grams of L-xylulose in the urine each day. The syndrome may give rise to the mistaken diagnosis of diabetes mellitus, but those individuals with the genetic defect causing pentosuria have not been shown to have any abnormality in glucose metabolism.

73. The answer is A. *(Stanbury, ed 3. p 1552.)* Renal tubular acidosis is characterized by a low concentration of serum bicarbonate and an approximately commensurate elevation in serum chloride.

74. The answer is A. *(Stanbury, ed 3. p 1556.)* The primary defect in renal tubular acidosis appears to be an inability of the distal tubule to generate steep pH gradients between blood and tubular urine. This is best explained by excessive back-diffusion of secreted hydrogen from urine to blood.

75. The answer is D. *(Stanbury, ed 3. p 1115.)* Intermittent acute porphyria does not result in cutaneous photosensitivity. Abdominal pain is the initial and often most prominent symptom. Acute attacks may vary in duration from several days to several months. Death in this disease is usually due to respiratory paralysis, but uremia and cachexia may contribute.

76. The answer is A. *(Davis, ed 2. pp 695-700.)* The rough or unencapsulated strains of *Diplococcus pneumoniae* are not thought to be pathogenic for humans. A capsule protects the bacteria and confers pathogenicity; the degree of virulence varies among antigenic types. Testing encapsulated species, e.g., type 3, with the appropriate antiserum leads to a positive quellung test (capsular swelling or refractivity).

77. The answer is C. *(Davis, ed 2. pp 758, 769.)* Mucoid colonies are typical of *Klebsiella* as is the lack of motility. *Proteus* and *Salmonella* are almost always motile. The ability to form butylene glycol (a positive Voges-Proskauer test) is typical of *Klebsiella* but of none of the other bacteria mentioned. *E. coli* and *P. vulgaris* are indole-positive. The negative ornithine reaction is typical but not specific for *K. pneumoniae*.

78. The answer is C. *(Davis, ed 2. p 459.)* T lymphocytes do not secrete IgG as do the plasma cells, which differentiates them from B lymphocytes. Rather, T lymphocytes may help or suppress functions of B lymphocytes or of other effector lymphocytes. T lymphocytes comprise the majority of lymphocytes in the immediate subcapsular and mantle zones surrounding follicles in lymph nodes, as well as in the periarteriolar regions (white pulp) of the spleen.

79. **The answer is A.** *(Davis, ed 2. p 418.)* IgA is present in exocrine secretions where it exerts an antibacterial effect. The other immunoglobulins listed, as well as low levels of IgA, are found in the serum.

80. **The answer is E.** *(Davis, ed 2. pp 587-588.)* All of the diseases listed have autoimmune components. In Goodpasture's syndrome there is production and deposition of an antibody which cross-reacts with the renal and pulmonary capillary basement membranes with resultant damage and hemorrhage.

81. **The answer is B.** *(Davis, ed 2. p 559.)* Delayed-hypersensitivity reactions are mediated by T lymphocytes and other mononuclear cells. The reaction requires previous exposure to antigen, frequently a large protein, and takes from one to three days to fully develop.

82. **The answer is A.** *(Davis, ed 2. p 549.)* Serum sickness is associated with antigen-antibody complexes produced and cleared in an environment of antigen excess. The complexes induce focal vascular lesions in many arterial and capillary beds. The other "allergic" responses listed are associated with much smaller amounts of antigen.

83. **The answer is C.** *(Davis, ed 2. pp 182-186.)* During transduction, a DNA-carrying phage enters or becomes associated with a bacterium. The DNA fragment enters the cell and is incorporated into its genetic pool. Transformation does not require the phage as mediator. Conjugation is also not phage-mediated. Transcription and recombination are events in nucleic acid synthesis.

84. **The answer is C.** *(Davis, ed 2. pp 1233, 1281.)* Picornaviruses, a class of small, icosahedral, single-stranded RNA viruses, include polioviruses, coxsackieviruses (aseptic meningitis and herpangina), the rhinoviruses (common cold), and the echoviruses (viral meningitis). The etiologic agent of keratoconjunctivitis is the type 8 adenovirus, an icosahedral, double-stranded DNA virus.

85. **The answer is D.** *(Davis, ed 2. pp 793-794.)* Aerobic growth of *H. influenzae* requires a rich medium that includes two growth factors known as X factor and V factor. X factor is heat-stable while V factor is not. *Staphylococcus aureus* can grow on the heat-treated chocolate agar and as a growth product produces V factor (NAD or NADP) which allows *H. influenzae* to grow near by. This phenomenon is called satellite phenomenon. The other four organisms listed are capable of growth in the absence of V factor.

86. The answer is E. *(Davis, ed 2. pp 845-847, 852-858.)* *M. tuberculosis* is an obligate aerobe, thus its predilection for pulmonary infection. The high content of lipids in its cell wall is in part responsible for its acid-fast response to Ziehl-Neelsen staining. The frequency of drug-resistant mutants in this organism has necessitated simultaneous use of multiple chemotherapeutic agents against it. Individuals with silicosis have a high incidence of infection with *M. tuberculosis*, which on culture requires several weeks to grow.

87. The answer is D. *(Davis, ed 2. pp 985-997.)* *C. neoformans* is a true pathogen. It is not dimorphic as are *C. immitis, H. capsulatum,* and *B. dermatitidis.* *A. fumigatus* is also not dimorphic, but grows as a mycelium and not as an encapsulated yeast. All of the organisms listed can cause systemic disease, but except for *C. neoformans*, respiratory involvement is their major clinical problem. Although *C. neoformans* usually enters via the lung, pulmonary involvement is often minimal, and the meningeal involvement is the most serious common aspect of infection.

88. The answer is C. *(Davis, ed 2. pp 1240, 1309.)* Influenza is caused by small, RNA viruses, classified as myxoviruses. All of the other viral illnesses listed, are caused by herpesviruses. These are relatively large, double-stranded DNA viruses. Shingles and chickenpox are caused by a virus, herpes zoster, which is identical to varicella. Cytomegalovirus and EB virus cause the other two diseases.

89. The answer is A. *(Davis, ed 2. p 938.)* In diagnosing *M. pneumoniae*, the classic bedside test was the presence of cold agglutinins (antibodies reacting with red blood cells at 4°C but not at 37°C). This test is non-specific but can be suggestive of *M. pneumoniae* infection: The same is true for antistreptococcal MG antibodies. Specific tests are now available which measure antimycoplasmal titers in acute phase and convalescent serum, but these give retrospective identification. Culture growth is slow and the diagnosis of *M. pneumoniae* infection is largely one of suspicion and exclusion by the clinician.

90. The answer is A. *(Davis, ed 2. p 636.)* *Salmonella typhi,* like many gram-negative organisms, contains a powerful endotoxin as part of its cell wall. *S. typhi* does not produce an exotoxin, as do all of the other listed organisms.

91. The answer is B. *(Robbins, 1974. p 364.)* *Staphylococcus aureus* elaborates many powerful toxins and enzymes. Two of these are thought to contribute to the tendency of *S. aureus* to produce localized infections and abscesses: coagulase may cause local vascular thrombosis; a necrotizing exotoxin is probably responsible for the localized tissue necrosis.

92. **The answer is A.** *(Anderson, ed 6. p 394.)* The three nuclei indicated by the arrow contain viral inclusions. In this case, varicella virus was the infecting agent. The presence of microscopic foci of necrosis in numerous parenchymal organs in an infant with a skin rash is typical of this viral disease in the perinatal period.

93. **The answer is E (all).** *(Robbins, 1974. p 40.)* Coagulative necrosis consists of the transformation of a cell into an acidophilic opaque body with preservation of the basic cell shape and usually with loss of the nucleus. This pattern presumably results from denaturation of the cell's protein after cell death occurs. It may be seen in a variety of conditions including all of the ones mentioned.

94. **The answer is B (1, 3).** *(Robbins, 1974. pp 51-53.)* Dystrophic calcification, by definition, is calcification occurring in dead or dying tissues. It can, and often does, occur in the presence of normal serum calcium. Metastatic calcification occurs in healthy tissue and almost always reflects disordered calcium metabolism, most often hypercalcemia, due to any number of causes including hyperparathyroidism, systemic sarcoidosis, and milk-alkali syndrome.

95. **The answer is B (1, 3).** *(Robbins, 1974. p 77.)* The reticuloendothelial system consists of a dispersed system of phagocytic cells capable of taking up dyes or particles from the blood. These cells are most abundant in the spleen, liver, bone marrow, and lymph nodes, but are also present in the lung as alveolar macrophages. They can participate in inflammatory reactions and may form giant cells. Kupffer cells are the phagocytic cells which line liver sinusoids. Langhans' cells are multinucleated giant cells seen in granulomatous reactions. Heart-failure cells are large mononuclear cells that contain phagocytized hemosiderin granules and are found in the sputum or lungs of patients with chronic pulmonary congestion as the result of left-sided heart failure. Plasma cells are not considered to be a part of the reticuloendothelial system.

96. **The answer is D (4).** *(Anderson, ed 6. p 250.)* Generally, cells undergoing continuous mitosis, such as intestinal epithelium, are extremely radiosensitive. Cells in interphase such as those from normal liver, kidney, and skeletal muscle are usually resistant to radiation damage at the stated dose.

97. **The answer is B (1, 3).** *(Anderson, ed 6. pp 71-72.)* Intestinal lipodystrophy (Whipple's disease) is a rare disorder involving intestinal fat absorption, in which granulomatous inflammation of fat followed by fibrosis is seen. Sclerema neonatorum is an inflammatory disorder affecting newborn infants. Insulin lipodystrophy is not an inflammatory condition and steatopygia refers to excessive fat deposits in the buttocks.

98. **The answer is B (1, 3).** *(Robbins, 1974. pp 1064, 1269-1271.)* Fat cells can be damaged by enzymes as in acute pancreatitis, or by trauma as in fat necrosis of the breast. Released fatty acids combine with calcium (saponification) to form insoluble salts which precipitate in situ.

99. **The answer is E (all).** *(Robbins, 1974. p 291.)* Diseases that lead to continued tissue synthesis and breakdown may produce hyperuricemia and clinical gout because of the resulting increase in nucleic acid turnover. This form of secondary gout may be seen in polycythemia vera, myeloid metaplasia, chronic leukemia, extensive psoriasis, and sarcoidosis. Cytolytic drugs, used in the chemotherapy of cancer, may augment hyperuricemia. Decreased renal excretion of uric acid may also lead to secondary gout.

100. **The answer is D (4).** *(Robbins, 1974. p 586.)* Atherosclerosis is a progressive disease that begins early in life and is characterized by the formation of atheromatous plaques in the aorta and in medium and large arteries. The atheroma consists of a raised focal fibrofatty plaque within the intima. The plaque has a core of lipid and a covering fibrous cap. Plaques may be complicated by calcification, internal hemorrhages, ulceration, and thrombus formation.

101. **The answer is E (all).** *(Robbins, 1974. pp 276-280.)* Hemosiderin may be seen in pulmonary macrophages as a result of red blood cell breakdown in a chronically congested lung. In idiopathic hemochromatosis, hemosiderin deposition is frequently associated with cirrhosis, diabetes, and skin pigmentation. (The skin pigment is, however, melanin.) Excess iron intake may also lead to hemosiderin deposition.

102. **The answer is B (1, 3).** *(Robbins, 1974. p 484.)* Vitamin D deficiency results in inadequate serum phosphorous and calcium levels and therefore in the impaired deposition of these minerals into the osteoid matrix. Insufficient mineralization of osteoid leads to the creation of soft, easily deformed bones. In vitamin D deficiency there is no failure of osteoid formation, and this results in a relative excess of osteoid in bone.

103. **The answer is A (1, 2, 3).** *(Robbins, 1974. p 296.)* Seven well defined syndromes resulting from genetic defects in enzymes responsible for glycogen metabolism have been described. Six of these diseases, including von Gierke's, Pompe's and McArdle's, are associated with excess accumulation of glycogen. The seventh disease is characterized by a lack of glycogen. Patients with Tay-Sachs disease have excessive accumulations of a ganglioside.

104. **The answer is A (1, 2, 3).** *(Anderson, ed 6. p 187.)* The first three changes described in the question have been documented in women taking oral contraceptives. Liver changes are also described but consist of portal triad inflammatory reactions without necrosis or bile duct proliferation.

105. The answer is C (2, 4). *(Anderson, ed 6. pp 514-524.)* Vitamins B_1 and C are rapidly excreted from the body and do not accumulate in toxic amounts. Both vitamin A and vitamin D are toxic when taken in large doses. Vitamin A intoxication causes periosteal proliferation of bone, particularly of the ulnae, clavicles, and metatarsals. Vitamin D intoxication has three principal effects: hypercalcemia, metastatic calcification, and osteitis fibrosa.

106. The answer is C (2, 4). *(Anderson, ed 6. pp 503-504.)* A majority of patients with diffuse scleroderma are female and they are usually found to have elevated gamma globulin levels. Degeneration of collagen with involvement of the skin and gastrointestinal tract are characteristic features of the disease. Scleroderma remains a disease of unknown etiology, although much recent evidence suggests that it may be an immunologic disorder. The lack of constant correlation between serum antibody titers and the activity of the disease process has prompted investigation of a possible cell-mediated mechanism to explain the course of scleroderma.

107. The answer is B (1, 3). *(Robbins, 1974. p 249.)* Plasmacytomas secrete monoclonal immunoglobulins, resulting in an abnormal monoclonal "spike" in the gamma globulin region on immunoelectrophoresis. Free immunoglobulin light chains are also found in approximately 50 percent of affected patients. These light chains, or Bence Jones proteins, pass into the urine because of their low molecular weight.

108. The answer is A (1, 2, 3). *(Anderson, ed 6. p 372.)* Trachoma, a chronic, progressive disease of the conjunctiva and cornea is caused by *Chlamydia*. The other diseases listed are caused by rickettsiae. Chlamydiae are generally classed as members of the psittacosis-lymphogranuloma-trachoma group. These are not viruses by present definition, but are thought to be small intracellular bacteria. Unlike viruses, they possess RNA and DNA, rudimentary enzyme systems, and a cell wall similar to that of gram-negative bacteria. The rickettsiae are also regarded as more closely related to the bacteria because of their electron-microscopic structure, chemical composition, and their binary division.

109. The answer is E (all). *(Anderson, ed 6. pp 389-392, 394.)* Inclusions may be seen within cells in lesions produced by all the viruses mentioned in standard tissue sections, although a careful search is sometimes necessary. Viral inclusion bodies may occur in both the cytoplasm and the nucleus. They vary in size and shape, but most tend to be eosinophilic and may be surrounded by a clear zone. Electron microscopic examinations of viral inclusions support the idea that many inclusions contain virions at some developmental stage.

110. The answer is A (1, 2, 3). *(Robbins, 1974. p 130.)* The Epstein-Barr virus, a herpesvirus, has been isolated from cultured Burkitt lymphoma cells, and it has been identified in cases of infectious mononucleosis and nasopharyngeal carcinoma. EB virus is capable of infecting normal lymphoid cells in vitro and producing changes suggestive of malignant transformation, but it has not been proven to cause human cancer.

111. The answer is E (all). *(Robbins, 1974. p 83.)* A granuloma consists of a small collection of modified macrophages surrounded by a rim of mononuclear cells which are principally lymphocytes. The modified macrophages are called "epitheloid" because their abundant cytoplasm and plump appearance cause them to resemble epithelial cells. Giant cells are also often present. Granulomas are seen in all of the conditions mentioned.

112. The answer is E (all). *(Robbins, 1974. pp 146-147.)* Circulating, tumor-specific antibodies may assist in tumor destruction or may sometimes interfere with tumor killing by sensitized lymphocytes (so-called "blocking antibodies"). Depressed cellular immunity, as in immunosuppressed allograft recipients, leads to an increased incidence of cancer. The complex interaction between the humoral and cellular immune response to tumor neoantigens may prove to be of crucial importance in the progression of a cancer.

113-115. The answers are: 113-C, 114-B, 115-A. *(Robbins, 1974. pp 154-155.)* Certain tumors express fetal or embryonic antigens which can aid in their diagnosis. Other cancers characteristically cause an elevation in the serum level of certain enzymes, such as acid phosphatase in cancer of the prostate.

116-119. The answers are: 116-A, 117-A, 118-D, 119-D. *(Robbins, 1974. pp 209, 222-223.)* Thymus-dependent lymphocytes play a critical role in the rejection of allograft tissues and organs and in the tuberculin skin reaction (delayed hypersensitivity). Anaphylaxis and hay fever are due to the interaction of mast cell-bound IgE and antigen that results in the release of histamine and other vasoactive compounds such as serotonin and the kinins.

120-123. The answers are: 120-D, 121-C, 122-B. 123-A. *(Robbins, 1974. p 203.)* The majority of the circulating gamma globulins in man are of the IgG class. IgE mediates allergic reactions by fixation to mast cells. IgM appears first in phylogeny and ontogeny, and is the first immunoglobulin secreted after initial antigen encounter. IgA contains a secretory piece, and is the major immunoglobulin present in secretions, such as tears and mucus.

Hematology

124. The answer is E. *(Beeson, ed 13. p 1518. Wintrobe, ed 7. p 1639.)* Early manifestations of a mismatched blood transfusion can include restlessness, anxiety, flushing of the face, precordial oppression and pain, tachycardia, tachypnea, and pain in the back and thighs. Shock may follow. A hemorrhagic tendency can develop immediately after the transfusion causing blood to ooze from the site of transfusion, the mucous membranes, or an operative site. This hemorrhagic tendency is due to the release of thromboplastic substances from red cells lysed intravascularly. This results in fibrin formation and depletion of fibrinogen and other labile clotting factors. The bleeding tendency may be the only sign in an anesthetized patient.

125. The answer is C. *(Wintrobe, Hematology, ed 7. p 1447. Williams, 1972. pp 17, 19.)* Auer bodies are cytoplasmic collections of nonspecific granules produced by immature myeloid leukocytes. They may be found in blast forms in acute myelogenous and myelomonoblastic leukemia. Döhle bodies stain bluish with Wright's stain and can be found in patients with severe infections, burns, or in association with the Chédiak-Higashi syndrome. Howell-Jolly bodies are remnants of nuclear chromatin and are commonly seen in the erythrocytes of patients with megaloblastic anemia, hemolytic anemia, or after splenectomy. Pappenheimer bodies are inorganic iron-containing granules occasionally seen in red cells stained with Wright's stain.

126. The answer is A. *(Wintrobe, Hematology, ed 7. pp 568-569.)* Normal, mature neutrophils have from two to five nuclear lobes; the polymorphonuclear neutrophil shown has at least six lobes. Hypersegmentation (the presence of more than five lobes) occurs in association with folic acid or vitamin B_{12} deficiency. The two deficiencies are also associated with macrocytic red cells and cannot be differentiated on the basis of the morphology of peripheral smears.

127. The answer is A. *(Williams, 1972. pp 28, 251.)* The cell in question is much larger than the other red cells, and has an immature nucleus with coarse, clumped chromatin. These features help to identify it as a nucleated red cell exhibiting megaloblastic maturation. The cell might be confused with a plasma cell, but plasma cells exhibit clumped chromatin which stains a dark purple, a deep blue cytoplasm, and nuclei which are small, eccentric, and often lie next to perinuclear clear zones.

128. The answer is B. *(Wintrobe, Hematology, ed 7. p 238.)* The cells shown in the photograph have a high nucleus to cytoplasm ratio, large nucleoli, very fine nuclear chromatin patterns, indented and/or folded nuclei, and grayish translucent cytoplasms. These characteristics are most consistent with monoblasts, and the cells shown exhibit "monocytoid" features. It is often difficult to differentiate types of blasts on a cytologic basis, especially monoblasts from myeloblasts. The smear shown is from a pure monoblastic leukemia.

129. The answer is E. *(Davidsohn, ed 15. p 126.)* Calcium pyrophosphate dihydrate, calcium oxalate monohydrate and monosodium urate crystals have a similar appearance in joint fluid. Calcium pyrophosphate dihydrate crystals exhibit weakly positive birefringence, while the other two exhibit negative birefringence. Talcum powder and cholesterol crystals exhibit birefringence, but can be identified by their nonneedle-like appearance. Calcium pyrophosphate dihydrate crystals are found in the joint fluids of individuals with a disease clinically identical to gout but called pseudogout or chondrocalcinosis.

130. The answer is D. *(Wintrobe, Hematology, ed 7. p 1612.)* The marrow of a patient with multiple myeloma contains diffuse and focal infiltrates of often immature and pleomorphic plasma cells. Fine chromatin, large nucleoli, multiple nuclei, and various inclusions can be found in myeloma plasma cells. Waldenström's macroglobulinemia marrow shows abnormal collections of immature lymphocytes. Erythroleukemia usually exhibits more mature erythroid forms in the marrow and peripheral blood and, of course, the typical abnormal myeloma protein is absent.

131. The answer is E. *(Davidsohn, ed 15. p 216.)* The photograph shown demonstrates the results of a sickling test for evaluation of the presence of hemoglobin S. The test does not differentiate homozygous from heterozygous states. Red cells that contain large amounts of normal or abnormal hemoglobins other than S rarely exhibit sickling. The test is based on the fact that erythrocytes containing a large proportion of hemoglobin S sickle in solutions of low oxygen content. Metabisulfite is a reducing substance which enhances the process of deoxygenation.

132. The answer is C. *(Anderson, ed 6. pp 1376, 1749.)* The eccentric nuclei and paranuclear halos are characteristic of plasma cells. Morphologically atypical features include marked size variation, binucleation and prominent nucleoli. Although these findings suggest a diagnosis of plasma cell dyscrasia (multiple myeloma), demonstration of a monoclonal immunoglobulin in the serum or concentrated urine would be required to confirm the diagnosis.

133. The answer is D. *(Davidsohn, ed 15. p 210.)* The sedimentation rate is characteristically low in sickle cell anemia due to the inhibition of rouleau formation produced by sickling of red blood cells. The anemia reflects the shortened red cell life span; Erythrocytes that contain 80 to 100 percent S hemoglobin have a life span approximately 25 percent of normal. Fetal hemoglobin appears to be heterogenously distributed among erythrocytes. The overall blood Hb F level may be as high as 20 to 25 percent, but this reflects the fact that some red cells contain as much as 50 percent Hb F.

134. The answer is C. *(Robbins, 1974. p 708.)* The abnormal chain in sickle cell hemoglobin is the beta chain and is designated β^S. The alpha chains are normal in both sickle cell disease and trait; an α^S allele does not exist. Individuals with a normal adult hemoglobin would be $\alpha\alpha\beta\beta$; people with sickle cell disease would be $\alpha\alpha\beta^S\beta^S$; therefore, individuals with sickle trait would be $\alpha\alpha\beta\beta^S$. Some individuals may inherit more than one genetic mutation, and thus produce not only hemoglobin S but hemoglobin C, D, or another abnormal hemoglobin. The genotype for these individuals would be written to reflect such combined defects.

135. The answer is D. *(Williams, 1972. pp 991-992. Anderson, ed 6. p 1813.)* The cell shown is characteristic of Gaucher's disease. The only other cell it might be confused with occurs in Niemann-Pick disease. In Niemann-Pick disease, however, the patients usually die within the first decade of life and histologically the cytoplasm is bubbly or foamy rather than striated.

136. The answer is B. *(Williams, 1972. pp 991-992.)* Inheritance of Gaucher's disease is most consistent with an autosomal recessive pattern. The disease appears to have a predilection for Ashkenazic Jews.

137. The answer is C. *(Williams, 1972. pp 676-677, 695-697.)* The sinusoids contain erythrocyte and myeloid precursors as well as maturing megakaryocytes. The absence of steatosis, necrosis, extensive polymorphonuclear infiltrate, and alcoholic hyalin excludes alcoholic hepatitis. The absence of necrosis, fibrous banding and bile stasis excludes viral hepatitis, cirrhosis, and extrahepatic biliary obstruction.

138. The answer is E. *(Williams, 1972. pp 676-677.)* The section shown was taken from a patient with severe myelofibrosis. Extramedullary hematopoiesis results from chronic destruction of the bone marrow. Myelomonocytic leukemia is an acute disease while porphyria, hemosiderosis and rheumatoid arthritis do not destroy normal bone marrow.

139. The answer is C. *(Williams, 1972. pp 270-272, 369.)* The megaloblastic anemia seen in alcoholic patients is almost always caused by decreased dietary intake of folic acid. Body folic acid stores may be depleted in a few months, whereas vitamin B_{12} stores last for several years. The megaloblastic anemias due to the other listed causes are usually associated with B_{12} deficiency.

140. The answer is C. *(Williams, 1972. p 1223.)* Clotting factor VIII is probably produced at several sites in the body; its production is not vitamin K dependent. The other four coagulation factors listed are produced in the liver, and their production is vitamin K dependent. Acquired disorders of the vitamin K-dependent coagulation factors are generally the result of liver dysfunction, abnormal absorption of vitamin K from the gastrointestinal tract, or the use of anticoagulant drugs.

141. The answer is A. *(Williams, 1972. p 1017.)* Prostaglandin E inhibits platelet aggregation, probably by increasing cyclic AMP levels within the platelets, while all the other agents listed promote it. Other potent inhibitors of platelet aggregation include mercurials and chemicals which react with sulfhydryl groups.

142. The answer is D. *(Williams, 1972. p 156.)* In vivo studies of chromium nuclide-tagged red blood cells show the normal red blood cell's life span to be about 120 days. In a disease state, the red cell life span may be finite, i.e., almost all cells will have approximately the same life span, or the red cells may undergo random destruction without regard to their age.

143. The answer is C. *(Williams, 1972. p 468.)* Complement-dependent erythrocyte lysis in acidified serum is relatively specific for paroxysmal nocturnal hemoglobinuria. The hemolytic uremic and Goodpasture syndrome are microangiopathic hemolytic disorders with an immunologic base. Pyruvate kinase deficiency and acute intermittent porphyria do not show this type of erythrocyte lysis. The acidified serum test is also referred to as the Ham test.

144. The answer is D. *(Williams, 1972. p 1217.)* While patients with von Willebrand's disease may exhibit hemarthrosis or spontaneous joint bleeding, these events occur much less frequently than in classic hemophilia and rarely lead to permanent joint deformities. Factor VIII levels and platelet adhesiveness are usually decreased in this disease. Menorrhagia is a common clinical finding in affected women.

145. The answer is E. *(Williams, 1972. p 1375.)* Of the conditions listed, only hereditary spherocytosis is associated with increased osmotic fragility. The other diseases generally have decreased red cell osmotic fragility. Autoincubation (24 hours at $37^{\circ}C$) increases the osmotic fragility of normal erythrocytes and that of red cells from patients with hereditary spherocytosis is increased to an even greater extent.

146. The answer is A. *(Williams, 1972. p 356.)* Delta-aminolevulinic acid (ALA) is a precursor in heme biosynthesis. Lead inhibits enzymes leading to heme synthesis and so increases delta-ALA levels in the body and excreted in the urine.

147. The answer is A. *(Williams, 1972. p 1258.)* Heparin does not interfere with the synthesis of vitamin K dependent coagulation factors. Coumarin exerts its anticoagulant action by inhibiting the hepatic production of factors II, VII, IX, and X, the vitamin K dependent factors. Heparin does, however, inhibit thrombin, factor Xa, and some platelet functions, and it increases fibrinolysis.

148. The answer is C. *(Williams, 1972. p 31.)* Chronic myelogenous leukemia is associated with a chromosomal abnormality, i. e., the Philadelphia chromosome, the deletion of an arm of chromosome 22. When abnormal chromosomes have been noted in other myeloproliferative disorders, the chromosome change has not been a constant one. However, involvement of the group C chromosomes seems to be most common.

149. The answer is C. *(Williams, 1972. p 920.)* The patient discussed has Hodgkin's disease in two separate lymph node groups in regions on the same side of the diaphragm and is, therefore, stage II. The systemic symptoms define the proper staging as II B. Stage I implies disease limited to one anatomic region, or two contiguous anatomic regions, on the same side of the diaphragm. Stage III is used to designate disease on both sides of the diaphragm but not extending beyond lymph nodes, spleen, and Waldeyer's ring. Stage IV is reserved for advanced disease present in tissues outside the Stage III lymphoreticular group. The subclasses A and B designate either the absence (A) or presence (B) of systemic symptoms in the individual patient.

150. The answer is E. *(Williams, 1972. p 947.)* Large lymphocytic-appearing cells with highly convoluted nuclei may appear in the peripheral blood of patients with mycosis fungoides. These cells, or similar appearing cells, may also be found in patients with lymphosarcoma and chronic lymphocytic leukemia. The skin lesions of mycosis fungoides are unique to that disorder and with the presence of Sézary cells confirm a diagnosis.

151. The answer is B. *(Williams, 1972. p 968.)* Whereas multiple myeloma may include all of the findings listed, the marrow of a patient with Waldenström's macroglobulinemia will contain predominantly lymphocytic-appearing infiltrates. Large numbers of plasma cells would strongly indicate a diagnosis of multiple myeloma rather than Waldenström's disease.

152. The answer is D. *(Williams, 1972. p 685.)* The leukocyte alkaline phosphatase (LAP) level is generally low in chronic granulocytic leukemia, while in the other listed disease states it is normal to elevated. The decrease in LAP can be documented by either histochemical or biochemical techniques. Remissions of chronic granulocytic leukemia may be signaled by increased LAP levels.

153. The answer is B. *(Williams, 1972. p 126.)* Normal serum iron levels range around 100 µg/100 ml and normal transferrin levels are approximately 300 ug/100 ml. Therefore, approximately 33 percent iron saturation of transferrin is usually found. Increased saturation occurs in hemochromatosis, while decreased saturation is present in iron deficiency anemia.

154. The answer is D. *(Davidshohn, ed 15. p 123. Williams, 1972. p 333.)* Both thalassemia minor and iron deficiency anemia are microcytic disorders in which affected patients' mean corpuscular hemoglobin usually is found to be reduced. Red blood cell indices may be useful to differentiate the two disorders, for while the mean corpuscular hemoglobin concentration is often normal or only slightly reduced in association with thalassemia minor, it is often definitely reduced in association with iron deficiency anemia. Both pernicious and folate deficiency anemias lead to megaloblastic changes in erythrocytes.

155. The answer is A. *(Williams, 1972. p 684.)* In chronic myelogenous leukemia (CML), the platelet count is often elevated rather than depressed. The other findings listed are typical of CML. In the one-third or more of CML patients with thrombocytosis, the peripheral blood may even show fragments of megakaryocyte nuclei.

156. The answer is E. *(Williams, 1972. p 391.)* Individuals with glucose 6-phosphate dehydrogenase (G6PD) deficiency may have acute hemolytic episodes when exposed to a variety of medications, including primaquine. In the other abnormalities listed, hemolysis is precipitated by other causes. The exact mechanism of erythrocyte hemolysis caused by drug administration is not known: It is accompanied by the formation of Heinz bodies, which are fragments of denatured protein, usually formed only in the presence of oxygen. Some of the hemolytic drugs form hydrogen peroxide during combination with hemoglobin; others form free radicals which also allow oxidation.

157. The answer is C. *(Williams, 1972. p 641.)* Felty's syndrome includes arthritis, splenomegaly and neutropenia. The other listed conditions are usually associated with neutrophilia. Acquired immunoneutropenia, associated with circulating autoantibody or leukotoxic factor, has been linked with connective tissue disease, monocytic leukemia, and some bone marrow disturbances.

158. The answer is B. *(Williams, 1972. p 566.)* The findings given are consistent with Wiskott-Aldrich syndrome. The Pelger-Hüet anomaly involves leukocytes with dumbbell-shaped nuclei: The leukocytes function normally. Chédiak-Higashi syndrome has some of the listed clinical features, but delayed hypersensitivity reactions are normal. In chronic granulomatous disease, leukocytes are unable to kill phagocytized bacteria, but delayed hypersensitivity reactions and platelet counts are normal. Hodgkin's disease presents a different constellation of symptoms.

159. The answer is C. *(Robbins, 1974. pp 778-779.)* Trauma is by far the most common cause of splenic rupture. Much less commonly, spontaneous rupture may occur in infectious mononucleosis, malaria, typhoid fever, leukemia, and other types of acute splenitis.

160. The answer is B (1, 3). *(Robbins, 1974. pp 760-761.)* The diagnosis of Hodgkin's disease depends on the total histologic picture and the presence of Reed-Sternberg cells. Reed-Sternberg-like cells may also be seen in infectious mononucleosis, mycosis fungoides and other conditions.

161. The answer is B (1, 3). *(Robbins, 1974. p 226.)* Erythrocytes coated with antierythrocyte antibodies are phagocytized more readily by the reticuloendothelial system. They also may be lysed directly by complement.

162. The answer is B (1, 3). *(Williams, 1972. p 251.)* Macrocytes and hypersegmented neutrophils result from a defect in nuclear maturation within the marrow and are common features of megaloblastic anemia. Myeloblasts would not be seen and anemia, not polycythemia, would be present.

163. The answer is A (1, 2, 3). *(Williams, 1972. pp 251-252.)* The megaloblastic cells shown are larger than normal erythroid precursors and do not show nuclear maturation. They are found in erythroleukemia with myeloblasts, pernicious anemia, dietary folate and B_{12} deficiencies, and in patients treated with antimetabolite therapy. Megaloblastic anemias responsive to B_1, B_6, and C, but not to A, have been reported.

164. The answer is E (all). *(Williams, 1972. pp 251-252.)* Although frequently more pronounced in the erythroid series, megaloblastic changes and nuclear abnormalities occur in the myeloid series including megakaryocytes. A drop in the M/E ration and an increased mitotic rate represent a response to the anemia.

165. The answer is C (2, 4). *(Williams, 1972. p 972.)* The substance shown is amyloid with characteristic staining and polarized light appearance. In so-called primary distribution, it is found in 8 to 12 percent of patients with multiple myeloma and usually involves all of the tissues mentioned. Amyloid deposition to this degree is uncommon in the tongue of elderly people. Primary amyloidosis accompanying multiple myeloma is most often associated with depression of normal immunoglobulin levels.

166. The answer is C (2, 4). *(Williams, 1972. p 974.)* Serum electrophoresis usually shows only decreased normal immunoglobulins and albumin. Urine electrophoresis followed by immunoelectrophoresis, in contrast, usually reveals a monoclonal spike. Rectal and joint biopsies stained with Congo red and viewed in polarized light are helpful in diagnosis. Dye absorption rates and total dye consumption from the circulation are unreliable.

167. The answer is E (all). *(Williams, 1972. p 972.)* Primary amyloidosis, which is associated with plasma cell dyscrasia, can lead to deposits in all of the tissues mentioned and produce the symptoms described.

168. The answer is A (1, 2, 3). *(Robbins, 1974. p 713. Williams, 1972. p 467.)* In patients with paroxysmal nocturnal hemoglobinuria iron may be lost either in the form of hemoglobin or hemosiderin in the urine. A hypercoagulable state with frequent arterial and venous thromboses may also occur. Acute leukemia may develop simultaneously, or in patients who have had paroxysmal nocturnal hemoglobinuria for several years.

169. The answer is E (all). *(Robbins, 1974. p 780.)* Splenomegaly may be produced by increased numbers of malignant cells, inflammatory cells, cells containing abnormal material (Gaucher's cells), and by congestion, as in portal hypertension.

170-174. The answers are: 170-B, 171-E, 172-E, 173-C, 174-D. *(Williams, 1972. pp 19, 30-31, 684-686, 717, 880-887, 1236.)* Auer rods are sharply outlined reddish rods in immature cells in acute myelogenous (granulocytic) or monocytic leukemias. Approximately 90 percent of patients with chronic myelogenous leukemia have the Philadelphia chromosome. This Ph[1] chromosome is present in the neoplastic cells. Leukocyte alkaline phosphatase activity is frequently very low. While high peripheral counts are common to all leukemias, none shows the variety of cells seen in chronic myelogenous leukemia. Unless the terminal blast crisis has occurred, myeloblasts may be relatively few. Acute promyelocytic leukemia often presents with widespread petechiae and ecchymoses from diffuse intravascular coagulation. Chronic lymphocytic leukemia occurs most frequently in the geriatric population (90 percent of cases occur in patients over the age of 50) and often does not require antimetabolite therapy for prolonged periods of time.

Cardiovascular System

175. The answer is A. *(Robbins, 1974. p 649.)* For many years it has been thought that ulceration or fracture of an atheromatous plaque, or hemorrhage into a plaque, was responsible for coronary artery thrombosis. Such thrombosis was thought to lead to coronary occlusion and myocardial infarction. Recently, however, it has been suggested that thrombi might be the result of acute myocardial infarction rather than the cause. In support of this contention, recent studies have demonstrated coronary artery thrombosis in less than 50 percent of the cases of myocardial infarction. The controversy has not yet been resolved.

176. The answer is E. *(Lehninger, 1970. p 355. Robbins, 1974. p 611.)* Raynaud's disease is characterized by episodic vasoconstriction of the small arteries and arterioles of the extremities. Cold weather aggravates the vasospasm which most commonly affects the fingers, hands, feet, and tip of the nose. Gangrene may develop in severe cases.

177. The answer is A. *(Robbins, 1974. p 336.)* Stasis of blood in fibrillating atria predisposes to thrombosis and embolism. Systemic embolization from left atrial thrombi may cause infarction in the brain, lower extremities, spleen, and kidneys.

178. The answer is C. *(Robbins, 1974. p 335.)* Ninety-five percent of pulmonary emboli arise from thrombi in the leg veins. Endothelial alterations, stasis or turbulence of blood flow, and increased blood coagulability may all contribute to vascular thrombosis.

179. The answer is D. *(Robbins, 1974. p 335.)* Most pulmonary emboli arise from thrombi in leg veins. Large emboli cause sudden death from systemic anoxia or acute right heart failure. Embolism in a patient without circulatory insufficiency may cause intra-alveolar hemorrhage but not infarction.

180. The answer is D. *(Robbins, 1974. p 616.)* Syphilitic aneurysms are almost always confined to the thoracic aorta and usually involve the ascending and transverse portions of the arch. The development of these aneurysms is based on the medial destruction characteristic of tertiary luetic aortitis. Atherosclerosis almost invariably develops in the thoracic aorta in the presence of syphilitic aortitis, and may contribute to the weakening of the wall.

181. The answer is A. *(Anderson, ed 8. p 402.)* Arteriosclerotic heart disease is characterized anatomically by atherosclerosis of the coronary arteries with consequent ischemic atrophy and fibrosis of the myocardium. These changes are frequently accompanied by degenerative fibrocalcific damage to the heart valves. Myocardial infarction results from sudden or relatively sudden arterial insufficiency. The photomicrograph illustrates infarction of the myocardium.

182. The answer is B. *(Robbins, 1974. p 651.)* By three days after a myocardial infarct, the predominant microscopic features include a marked exudate of neutrophils and coagulation necrosis of myocardial fibers. Grossly, the infarcted area appears pale with a hypertensive border.

183. The answer is D. *(Robbins, 1974. p 654.)* In myocardial infarction, life-threatening arrhythmias occur in approximately 45 percent of patients without shock and in more than 90 percent of patients with shock. The most common arrhythmias are ventricular, but atrial extrasystoles, sinus tachycardia, and sinus bradycardia also occur. Even without arrhythmias, nearly two-thirds of patients with acute myocardial infarcts develop heart failure and pulmonary edema. Sudden death (death within 24 hours of onset of symptoms) occurs in about 20 to 25 percent of acute attacks.

184. The answer is B. *(Robbins, 1974. p 650.)* Although all the signs mentioned in the question can occur, they are not inevitably present. There is not always a demonstrable coronary artery thrombus at autopsy: this is especially true in those patients who die shortly after the infarction.

185. The answer is C. *(Anderson, ed 6. pp 625-627.)* The photograph shows a spontaneous rupture of the posterior left ventricular wall. This is a recognized complication of acute myocardial infarct with myocardial cell necrosis. It occurs most often within two weeks of onset of infarction. The determining factors are the systolic intraventricular pressure and the degree of tissue softening. None of the other pathologic processes listed are generally associated with cardiac rupture.

186. The answer is B. *(Robbins, 1974. p 665.)* Carditis, chorea, erythema marginatum, subcutaneous nodules, and polyarthritis are the major diagnostic features of acute rheumatic fever. The presence of any two of these major Jones' criteria indicates a high probability of the presence of rheumatic fever.

187. The answer is A. *(Robbins, 1974. p 660.)* Endocardial involvement is the most serious aspect of rheumatic fever and causes most of the deaths, usually years after the acute disease has subsided. The mitral valve is almost always involved in rheumatic valvulitis, either alone or in combination with the aortic valve. Acute valvulitis consists of swelling of the valves with friable verrucae present along the lines of closure. Fibrous healing leads to thickening of the valves and stenosis.

188. The answer is A. *(Robbins, 1974. pp 657-666.)* Acute rheumatic carditis typically affects all three layers of the heart, but damage to the valves causes most of the subsequent deaths.

189. The answer is B. *(Hurst, ed 3. pp 613, 700.)* Rubella is a prototype of an environmental cause of congenital malformation. Cardiac defects, cataracts, microcephaly, mental retardation, and anomalies of dental structures may all be associated with maternal rubella infection. Patent ductus arteriosus is the most common cardiac defect occurring in congenital rubella. It is approximately three times more common than ventricular septal defect, which is the next most common cardiovascular finding. Atrial septal defects, pulmonary artery stenosis, and tetralogy of Fallot occur much less frequently.

190. The answer is A. *(Anderson, ed 6. p 663.)* Clinically significant pulmonary stenosis is rarely an acquired lesion. Most cases are congenital, occurring in conjunction with other cardiac anomalies.

191. The answer is B. *(Hurst, ed 3. p 1290.)* In congenital heart disease, ventricular septal defect is the lesion most often involved in bacterial endocarditis, accounting for approximately 50 percent of cases. It is followed in frequency by patent ductus arteriosus, pulmonic stenosis, and aortic stenosis.

192. The answer is D. *(Robbins, 1974. p 671.)* Systemic blood flow in the lesion described must come from the right heart through a patent ductus into the aorta in order for the patient to survive even briefly. Surgical correction must be done in the first year of life.

193. The answer is B. *(Robbins, 1974. pp 236-239.)* The focal inflammatory lesions of polyarteritis nodosa may affect any artery of medium or small size or any arteriole in any organ of the body. The lesions are characterized histologically by acute necrosis of the media with extension into the intima and destruction of the internal elastica. A heavy infiltrate of polymorphonuclear leukocytes and thrombosis of the vessel follow the acute necrosis. A remnant of the internal elastica is visible in the vessel pictured.

194. The answer is B (1, 3). *(Robbins, 1974. p 601.)* Mönckeberg's sclerosis consists of calcification of the media of muscular arteries. It affects both women and men, but rarely before the age of 50. The lesions can be produced in laboratory animals by infusions of such vasoconstrictors as nicotine and epinephrine. The medial calcification does not produce narrowing of the lumen.

195. The answer is C (2, 4). *(Robbins, 1974. pp 615-620.)* Dissecting aneurysms almost always occur in hypertensive patients whose aortas are weakened by cystic medial necrosis. Syphilis and arteriosclerosis may cause aneurysms, but they are classically not dissecting aneurysms.

196. The answer is D (4). *(Anderson, ed 6. pp 242, 611.)* The four symptoms mentioned in the question constitute the CRST (calcinosis, Raynaud's phenomenon, sclerodactyly, and telangiectasia) syndrome of scleroderma, and were originally considered to constitute a benign form of progressive systemic sclerosis. In the CRST syndrome, Raynaud's phenomenon is secondary to other pathology. Cold sensitivity of the fingers as a primary condition, i.e., without a causal disease, is termed Raynaud's disease.

197. The answer is B (1, 3). *(Robbins, 1974. p 683.)* The two most common agents that lead to constrictive pericarditis are staphylococci and the tubercle bacilli. The pericardial space is obliterated and transformed into a dense scar which may even be calcified. Nonsuppurative pericarditis, as seen in rheumatic fever or uremia, rarely leads to constrictive pericarditis.

198. The answer is B (1, 3). *(Robbins, 1974. p 651.)* Myocardial infarction results from sudden or relatively sudden coronary arterial insufficiency. Total occlusion of either the left anterior descending or the right coronary artery is found in 80 percent of cases, but the infarct almost invariably occurs in the left ventricle or interventricular septum.

199. The answer is B (1, 3). *(Robbins, 1974. p 661.)* Valves damaged by acute rheumatic fever contain irregular, warty vegetations along the lines of closure where the valves impinge on each other. These verrucae probably result from the precipitation of fibrin at sites of endothelial damage. Rheumatic valvulitis may lead to fibrous scarring and functional impairment.

200. The answer is B (1, 3). *(Robbins, 1974. pp 666-670.)* Shunting of blood from the right to the left side of the heart without passing through the lungs is necessary to produce cyanosis. The shunt in a patent ductus arteriosus or an atrial septal defect is from left to right. Transposition and tetralogy produce a right to left shunt.

201. The answer is C (2, 4). *(Anderson, ed 6. pp 658-660.)* Mitral stenosis is most often associated with aortic valve disease and occasionally with tricuspid valve disease especially in people with antecedent rheumatic fever. Occasionally both aortic and mitral disease result from atherosclerosis. Pulmonary valvular stenosis is rarely caused by either. Since severe mitral stenosis prevents significant regurgitation, left ventricular enlargement would not be expected. Left atrial enlargement and chronic pulmonary congestion are common in mitral disease.

202. The answer is A (1, 2, 3). *(Anderson, ed 6. p 719.)* The fourth anomaly associated with tetralogy of Fallot is a ventricular septal defect, not tricuspid insufficiency.

203. The answer is A (1, 2, 3). *(Robbins, 1974. pp 682-685.)* Serous and fibrinous pericarditis may occur in uremia, rheumatic fever, or myocardial infarction. They usually resolve without major sequellae. Purulent pericarditis, secondary to bacterial or viral infection, is much more serious and may lead to constrictive pericarditis.

204-207. The answers are: 204-A, 205-C, 206-D, 207-B. *(Robbins, 1974. pp 657-665, 682-686.)* Tuberculosis may spread from mediastinal nodes to the pericardium. Primary myocarditis is frequently caused by type B coxsackievirus or echoviruses. Rheumatic fever follows a streptococcal infection, and syphilis may cause aortic aneurysms, usually thoracic. *E. coli* forms part of the normal flora of the intestinal tract.

208-211; The answers are: 208-B, 209-A, 210-C, 211-D. *(Robbins, 1974. pp 657, 686-688.)* Aschoff bodies are granulomatous formations appearing in the proliferative phase of acute, rheumatic myocarditis. They consist of focal and diffuse cellular infiltrates including lymphocytes, macrophages, fibroblasts and multinucleated giant cells. They are pathognomonic for rheumatic myocarditis. Trypanosomiasis (Chagas' disease) involving the myocardium is common in parts of South America, accounting for over 75 percent of all heart disease in some localities. In its chronic form, it is associated with cardiac enlargement and arrhythmias. Acute, idiopathic (Fiedler's) myocarditis is also called giant cell myocarditis. A history of antecedent respiratory infection is common. Most cases occur in the third decade of life. Inflammatory lesions are limited to the myocardium. Viral invasion of the myocardium is seen in type B coxsackievirus infections in the young.

212-214. The answers are: 212-E, 213-B, 214-A. *(Robbins, 1974. pp 614-617.)* Congenital berry aneurysms usually affect the cerebral vessels. Ninety-seven percent of abdominal aneurysms are arteriosclerotic, and syphilitic aneurysms are virtually always confined to the thoracic aorta. Luetic aneurysms may also cause dilatation of the aortic valve or narrowing of the coronary ostium.

215-217. The answers are: 215-B, 216-A, 217-C. *(Robbins, 1974. pp 236-238, 586-607.)* The initial lesion in polyarteritis nodosa is fibrinoid necrosis of the media. This is followed by an intense inflammatory infiltrate that affects the entire vessel wall. Giant cells and a granulomatous reaction along the disrupted elastica interna characterize giant cell arteritis. Intimal lipid accumulation is an early atherosclerotic lesion.

Respiratory System

218. The answer is C. *(Robbins, 1974. p 828.)* The renal and pulmonary lesions of Goodpasture's syndrome are a consequence of antibodies that react with the basement membranes of the glomeruli and pulmonary septa. Uremia is the most common cause of death. Bilateral nephrectomy may lead to reversal of the pulmonary lesions.

219. The answer is C. *(Robbins,1974. p 797.)* Patients with homozygous antitrypsin deficiency develop severe panlobular emphysema, often before the age of 40. This genetic disorder accounts for about 10 percent of cases of emphysema. Other factors in the pathogenesis of emphysema include air pollution and smoking.

220. The answer is B. *(Robbins, 1974. pp 792-800.)* Emphysema is defined as a disease or group of diseases characterized by enlargement of air spaces distal to the terminal bronchioles with destruction of alveolar septa.

221. The answer is B. *(Robbins, 1974. pp 832-838.)* Bronchogenic carcinoma is the most common visceral malignancy in men, accounting for 40 percent of all male cancer deaths. Lung cancer is at least ten times as common in smokers as in nonsmokers. Bronchogenic carcinomas arise most often near the hilus of the lung, in the lower trachea, or first, second, or third order bronchi.

222. The answer is D. *(Robbins, 1974. p 803.)* Extrinsic or atopic asthma is most commonly triggered by environmental antigens such as dust, pollen, animal dander, and foods. Mast cells with bound IgE will release various vasoactive agents upon interaction with the sensitizing antigen.

223. The answer is A. *(Beeson, ed 13. p 919. Wintrobe, ed 7. p 1317.)* Byssinosis is a form of pneumoconiosis caused by the inhalation of cotton dust. "Monday dyspnea" in byssinosis is associated with decreases of FEV_1 (forced expiratory volume in 1 sec) of flow rates on MEFV (maximum expiratory flow/volume) curves, and with impairment of intrapulmonary mixing. Since isoproterenol reverses symptoms and function loss, the airway obstruction is probably caused by contraction of smooth muscles.

224. The answer is C. *(Hughes, 1968. p 104.)* Squamous metaplasia frequently occurs in response to irritation or infection. It is frequently seen in specimens of sputum from heavy smokers and patients with chronic respiratory infections. Metaplastic squamous cells are also frequently seen in patients with carcinoma of the lung, but they are not by themselves indicative of neoplasia.

225. The answer is E. *(Anderson, ed 6. pp 421-422.)* The Grocott (methenamine silver) stain shown emphasizes the pseudohyphae and yeast forms of *Candida* species. The pattern of vessel invasion is characteristic of many pathogenic fungi, including *Candida*. Such infections tend to occur in immunologically-suppressed patients with other severe, usually neoplastic diseases.

226. The answer is C. *(Anderson, ed 6. pp 446-447.)* The presence of oval and helmet-shaped organisms whose capsules take a silver stain within a foamy alveolar infiltrate in an individual with leukemia is diagnostic of *Pneumocystis carinii* infection. The organism usually is opportunistic, infecting severely ill, immunologically-depressed patients.

227. The answer is B. *(Anderson, ed 6. p 974. Beeson, ed 13. p 926.)* The common nonmetastatic endocrine manifestations seen in patients with bronchogenic carcinoma include inappropriate secretion of antidiuretic hormone, Cushing's syndrome, and hypercalcemia. Oat cell is the most common histologic type of carcinoma associated with these manifestations.

228. The answer is E. *(Anderson, ed 6. p 976.)* In some reported series of primary, malignant, pulmonary tumors arising in pre-existing scars, over 50 percent were adenocarcinomas.

229. The answer is B (1, 3). *(Robbins, 1974. pp 802-803, 833-838.)* Heavy cigarette smoking causes excessive mucus secretion, destruction of ciliary action, squamous metaplasia, and dysplasia. Smoking is one of the major etiologic factors in chronic bronchitis and in bronchogenic carcinoma.

230. The answer is E (all). *(Robbins, 1974. p 806.)* Bronchiectasis is a chronic necrotizing infection of the bronchi and bronchioles associated with abnormal dilatation of these airways. It is not clear whether obstruction leads to the dilatation and infection, or whether the infection is the primary lesion. Evidence for both hypotheses is provided by the associations of bronchiectasis with asthma, chronic sinusitis, avitaminosis A, and fibrocystic disease.

231. The answer is D (4). *(Robbins, 1974. p 40.)* Caseous necrosis is a distinctive combination of coagulative and liquefactive necrosis seen characteristically in the center of tuberculous granulomas. The capsule of *Mycobacterium tuberculosis* contains materials that denature proteins and split lipids, transforming dead cells into clumped, cheesy material.

232. The answer is E (all). *(Robbins, 1974. p 467.)* The most common cause of bilateral, asymptomatic, hilar lymphadenopathy is sarcoidosis. The enlarged hilar lymph nodes almost never calcify and generally regress over a period of time. Histologically, the granulomas of sarcoid are noncaseating, and in long-standing disease will show progressive collagenous fibrosis. However, other diseases may have associated non-necrotic granulomas, i.e., tuberculosis, berylliosis, and syphilis. The diagnosis of sarcoidosis should not be made until other diseases have been ruled out by appropriate tests.

233. The answer is E (all). *(Anderson, ed 6. p 903.)* All of the answers given are recognized complications of emphysema of long duration. The reason for the presence of peptic ulcer disease in approximately 20 percent of patients with chronic emphysema is unclear.

234. The answer is C (2, 4). *(Anderson, ed 6. pp 942-943.)* The morphologic features of usual interstitial pneumonia (UIP) include interstitial edema and edema with hyaline membrane formation within the small air spaces in early lesions. An infiltrate of monocytes and lymphocytes then occurs. Regenerating alveolar epithelium relines damaged alveoli by "growing over" the alveolar exudate and thus incorporates this material into the interstitium. Fibrosis follows and may produce a pattern of randomly communicating air spaces lined by fibrous walls and metaplastic epithelium referred to as "honeycomb lung." Many people with UIP survive for many years. There is no described increase in the incidence of primary malignancy.

235. The answer is E (all). *(Anderson, ed 6. pp 944-946.)* All of the agents mentioned produce interstitial fibrosis if given in sufficient quantity over an extended period of time. Investigators have shown that the interstitial fibrosis associated with busulfan may be the result of organization of intra-alveolar fibrin and edematous fluid, with subsequent incorporation into the interalveolar septa. Reported oxygen damage is related to the concentration of oxygen and the duration of exposure. The response of the lung to these agents may represent a reaction that can follow pulmonary injury caused by several different agents.

236. The answer is C (2, 4). *(Robbins, 1974. pp 818-820.)* The initial lesion in primary tuberculosis consists of a focus of infection in the subpleural parenchyma, near the interlobar fissure, and infection of the draining regional nodes. These lesions usually resolve spontaneously.

237. **The answer is E (all).** *(Anderson, ed 6. pp 974-975.)* All of the systemic symptoms and syndromes mentioned occur in conjunction with bronchogenic carcinomas of various histologic types. The most common endocrine manifestation is probably Cushing's syndrome but the number and variety of tumor-associated endocrine syndromes has increased dramatically in recent years. Additional neuromuscular abnormalities associated with lung tumors include mental status changes ranging from impaired acuity to dementia, degenerative myopathy, and a myasthenia gravis-like syndrome.

238. **The answer is D (4).** *(Anderson, ed 6. p 893.)* The photomicrograph shows classic hyaline membranes coating alveolar sacs and ducts and is diagnostic of the respiratory distress syndrome of the newborn.

239. **The answer is E (all).** *(Anderson, ed 6. p 893.)* The presence of hyaline membranes indicates a diagnosis of acute alveolar injury which can occur in all of the conditions mentioned.

240. **The answer is B (1, 3).** *(Robbins, 1974. pp 786-789.)* Pulmonary emboli cause infarction in patients with compromised cardiovascular function. Those individuals with sufficient circulation are protected against pulmonary infarction by the bronchial artery blood supply to the pulmonary parenchyma. Parenchymal hemorrhage, but not infarction, will occur in these circumstances. The diagnostic features are ischemic necrosis of the lung parenchyma with hemorrhage. Such infarcts eventually organize with scar formation.

241-244. **The answers are: 241-D, 242-A, 243-B, 244-C.** *(Robbins 1974. pp 809-829.)* Acute left heart failure causes pulmonary edema. Excessive use of oily nose drops may cause lipid pneumonia with accumulation of lipid within alveolar macrophages. Goodpasture's syndrome may present as hemoptysis secondary to necrotizing hemorrhagic interstitial pneumonitis. Histologically, the alveoli are filled with blood. The alveoli in acute bronchopneumonia are filled with an exudate of polymorphonuclear leukocytes.

245-248. **The answers are: 245-B, 246-D, 247-C, 248-A.** *(Robbins, 1974. pp 832-845.)* The squamous cell carcinoma is the most common type of bronchogenic carcinoma. It arises from bronchial lining cells. Alveolar cell carcinomas arise from alveolar or bronchiolar lining cells. Mesotheliomas arise from the pleural lining cells. The adenoid cystic carcinoma resembles the adenoid cystic carcinoma of the salivary glands, supporting the idea that they arise from glandular epithelium in the bronchi.

Gastrointestinal System

249. The answer is A. *(Robbins, 1974. pp 924-927.)* Ten percent of patients with pernicious anemia and its associated atrophic gastritis may be expected to develop gastric carcinoma. Impaired DNA synthesis, from the vitamin B_{12} deficiency, has been postulated to play a role in this pathogenesis of gastric carcinoma.

250. The answer is A. *(Robbins, 1974. pp 935-939.)* Regional enteritis primarily affects the ileum, but other areas of the intestinal tract may also be involved. Crohn's disease is characterized by segmental areas of involvement which are sharply demarcated from the contiguous normal gut. The intestinal wall is thickened with chronic inflammatory cells and fibrosis affecting all layers. Noncaseating granulomas are frequently present.

251. The answer is C. *(Robbins, 1974. pp 946-947.)* Primary bowel diseases (sprue and celiac disease) and deficient secretions of enzymes or bile (pancreatic insufficiency or biliary obstruction) can cause malabsorption. Villous adenomas may occasionally produce excessive electrolyte losses, but not true malabsorption.

252. The answer is D. *(Robbins, 1974. pp 917-923.)* Duodenal ulcers are thought to be the consequence of the destructive action of increased acid-peptic secretions. These ulcers are much more common in men, and a disproportionately large number of affected patients have blood group O.

253. The answer is C. *(Robbins, 1974. p 976.)* Tumors of the appendix are very rare. The most frequent is the argentaffinoma. Sixty percent of carcinoids occur in the appendix, where they may invade through the muscularis but virtually never metastasize. These small lesions rarely produce the carcinoid syndrome.

254. The answer is C. *(Robbins, 1974. p 641.)* Centrilobular congestion surrounded by paler, sometimes fatty, peripheral lobular parenchyma gives a "nutmeg" pattern secondary to chronic passive congestion. Severe congestion may cause hepatocyte necrosis and fibrosis.

255. The answer is C. *(Robbins, 1974. pp 956-960.)* Up to 33 percent of patients with chronic ulcerative colitis may develop carcinoma. The cancers develop, on an average, 16 years after onset of colitis. Cancer is found in a high percentage of villous adenomas, but polypoid adenomas are not premalignant.

256. The answer is D. *(Anderson, ed 6. pp 1201-1202.)* Acute alcoholic hepatitis can be superimposed on a liver with pre-existing fatty change, portal cirrhosis, or in a previously normal organ. Although portal cirrhosis may accompany, or follow, acute alcoholic hepatitis, its presence is not required for the diagnosis. The consistent microscopic findings include hepatocellular degeneration and necrosis, inflammatory cell infiltrates, sclerosis of centrilobular sinusoids, steatosis, and cholestasis. The presence of Mallory bodies in hepatocytes ringed by leukocytes is often of great diagnostic help.

257. The answer is C. *(Anderson, ed 6. p 1239.)* Almost half of all primary cancers metastasize to the liver, according to large autopsy series. No primary hepatic tumor, benign or malignant, approaches this incidence.

258. The answer is E. *(Anderson, ed 6. pp 450-454.)* The submucosal position in the distal colon, the history of residence in an endemic region, and the presence of spines as shown help to identify this parasite as one of three species of *Schistosoma*, in this case *mansoni*.

259. The answer is C. *(Robbins, 1974. p 1049.)* Gallstones are found in 65-95 percent of carcinomatous gallbladders. The etiology is unknown, but chronic inflammation and the known carcinogenic action of cholic acid derivatives might play a role. Most carcinomas have invaded the liver by the time they are discovered.

260. The answer is A. *(Robbins, 1974. p 1068.)* Sixty to seventy percent of carcinomas of the pancreas arise in the head of the pancreas. Because of their location, tumors of the head produce biliary obstruction relatively early and may thus be detected before widespread metastases have occurred. However, surgical cure of carcinoma of the pancreas is unusual regardless of location.

261. The answer is B. *(Ackerman, ed 5. pp 490-491.)* The lesion pictured is a basaloid or cloacogenic carcinoma that has the same gross appearance as the more common epidermoid carcinoma, but histologically resembles the basal cell carcinoma of the skin.

262. The answer is B. *(Ackerman, ed 5. p 524.)* Chronic hepatitis has been defined as an inflammatory process of the liver that lasts longer than one year and lacks the nodular regeneration and architectural distortion of cirrhosis. In chronic active hepatitis, an intense inflammatory reaction with numerous plasma cells spreads from portal tracts into periportal areas. It destroys the limiting plate and results in formation of periportal hepatocytic islets. The prognosis is poor, and the majority of patients develop cirrhosis. Chronic persistent hepatitis is usually a sequela of acute viral hepatitis. It has a benign course, without progression to chronic active hepatitis or cirrhosis. The portal inflammation does not extend into the periportal areas, thus differentiating it from chronic active hepatitis.

263. The answer is D. *(Robbins, 1974. pp 932-933.)* Meckel's diverticulum is a vestigial remnant of the omphalomesenteric duct and is usually found in the ileum, approximately 12 inches proximal to the ileocecal valve. One-half of these diverticula are found to contain heterotopic rests of gastric mucosa. Peptic ulceration in the adjacent intestinal mucosa may occur.

264. The answer is B (1, 3). *(Anderson, ed 6. p 1119.)* Congenital pyloric stenosis is seen predominantly in male infants at the age of approximately three weeks. It requires prompt surgical incision of the stenotic pyloric muscle.

265. The answer is A (1, 2, 3). *(Robbins, 1974. pp 952-953.)* Absence of ganglion cells from the myenteric plexus produces a segment of bowel where normal propulsive contraction can not occur, thus inducing a functional obstruction. The aganglionic segment itself is not distended, just the bowel proximal to it. The disease usually affects the rectum and rectosigmoid, but occasionally may affect the entire colon, and even part of the small intestine.

266. The answer is E (all). *(Robbins, 1974. pp 916-917.)* Acute gastric ulcers ("stress ulcers") may occur in a variety of situations. Those associated with head injury or intracranial surgery have been linked with increased gastric acid production. Corticosteroid therapy may qualitatively alter the gastric mucus production and decrease the turnover rate of gastric mucosa epithelium. Nearly all stress situations are linked with increased endogenous steroid production, so "stress ulcers" may be the result of steroid mechanisms. "Stress ulcers" are usually less than 1 cm in diameter and typically involve only the mucosa.

267. The answer is A (1, 2, 3). *(Beeson, ed 14. p 1209.)* The diarrhea associated with the Zollinger-Ellison syndrome is caused by massive gastric hypersecretion and can be relieved by nasogastric aspiration or by total gastrectomy. The large amount of acid produces mucosal damage and intestinal hypermotility. In addition, gastrin decreases salt and water absorption from the intestine. The diarrhea is frequently accompanied by steatorrhea which is caused by inactivation of pancreatic lipase, precipitation of conjugated bile salts at low intraluminal pH, and direct mucosal damage by the acid.

268. The answer is E (all). *(Robbins, 1974. p 924.)* Ten percent of patients with pernicious anemia and its associated atrophic gastritis and achlorhydria will develop cancer of the stomach. Benign gastric adenomatous polyps are also associated with an increased incidence of malignancy. There is evidence that an autoimmune disorder leads to atrophic gastritis. Pernicious anemia develops because of deficient intrinsic factor production by the atrophic gastric mucosa.

269. The answer is E (all). *(Robbins, 1974. pp 972-973.)* Common ulcerative lesions of the intestine seen in the United States include ulcerative colitis, tuberculous ulcers, uremic ulceration, and staphylococcal colitis following antibiotic therapy. Bacillary dysentery, cholera, and typhoid are common causes outside the U.S.

270. The answer is A (1, 2, 3). *(Robbins, 1974. p 947.)* Celiac disease is a form of hypersensitivity to the gliadin fraction of gluten. The characteristic anatomic finding is marked atrophy of the villi and microvilli of the jejunum. The clinical features of steatorrhea, diarrhea, weight loss, and malnutrition respond promptly to the removal of gluten from the diet.

271. The answer is D (4). *(Anderson, ed 6. pp 1120-1121.)* Diverticula occur most frequently in men over the age of 50, in the descending and sigmoid colon. The colon is the most commonly involved segment of the gastrointestinal tract. A majority of these lesions are not "true" diverticula, since the mucosa and muscularis mucosa herniate through defects in the muscular wall.

272. The answer is D (4). *(Robbins, 1974. pp 953-955.)* The pathogenesis of diverticulosis appears to be increased intraluminal pressure with eventual herniation of the mucosa and submucosa through the bowel wall. Whether congenital foci of muscular weakness pre-exist is uncertain, but the high frequency of diverticulosis in the general population argues against a specific congenital defect.

273. The answer is E. (all). *(Robbins, 1974. pp 973-975.)* Appendicitis is the most common cause of an acute "surgical" abdomen. It is most prevalent in young adults, and may be confused with a variety of conditions including all of those mentioned. The pathogenesis of acute appendicitis is poorly understood.

274. The answer is E (all). *(Anderson, ed 6. p 1127.)* Any disease state that increases pressure in the hemorrhoidal veins will produce or exacerbate hemorrhoids. All the listed entities will do this.

275. The answer is E (all). *(Robbins, 1974. p 989.)* Eighty-five percent of bilirubin is derived from the breakdown of red cells in the reticuloendothelial system. The heme pigment is ultimately converted into bilirubin, which is then taken up by the liver and conjugated to glucuronic acid. The water soluble bilirubin diglucuronide (conjugated) is secreted into the bile canaliculi. The process may be interfered with at any level, leading to jaundice.

276. The answer is E (all). *(Robbins, 1974. pp 990, 1033-1034.)* It is important to distinguish intrahepatic from extrahepatic obstructive jaundice, because the latter is often amenable to surgical treatment, as in biliary obstruction due to gallstones. Chronic unrelieved obstruction may lead to cirrhosis. Cellular swelling within the liver in viral hepatitis may lead to obstructive cholestasis and increased levels of conjugated bilirubin.

277. The answer is A (1, 2, 3). *(Robbins, 1974. p 1001.)* Centrilobular necrosis is usually the result of ischemia, and is most often associated with congestive cardiac failure. Centrilobular necrosis without congestion is typical of carbon tetrachloride and chloroform poisoning. Eclampsia and phosphorus poisoning characteristically produce peripheral necrosis, often with hemorrhage and sinusoidal thrombosis.

278. The answer is A (1, 2, 3). *(Robbins, 1974. p 997.)* Chronic passive congestion initially causes distension of the sinusoids with red cells. The mottled pattern of red dilated sinusoid surrounded by pale hepatic parenchyma is said to resemble a nutmeg. Centrilobular necrosis and fibrosis around the central veins may occur in chronic severe cases.

279. The answer is E (all). *(Ackerman, ed 5. p 527.)* Extrahepatic biliary obstruction due to stones in the common duct may lead to jaundice, ascending cholangitis, and gram-negative sepsis. Prompt operative intervention is indicated in order to remove the obstruction and prevent further sepsis. Liver biopsy may be helpful in chronic obstruction; in acute obstruction it may not serve to differentiate extrahepatic obstruction from intrahepatic cholestasis due to viral hepatitis, drug reactions, or other diseases.

280. The answer is E (all). *(Robbins, 1974. p 1005.)* Infectious hepatitis or hepatitis A is characterized by an acute onset relative to hepatitis B or serum hepatitis. Liver function usually returns to normal in 4 to 6 weeks, and fatalities are rare. Hepatitis B has a more unpredictable course, but the diseases are morphologically indistinguishable.

281. The answer is E (all). *(Ackerman, ed 5. p 531.)* Hepatic granulomas may be part of numerous pathologic processes including sarcoidosis, histoplasmosis and tuberculosis. Granuloma formation is a feature of primary biliary cirrhosis, and some patients with Hodgkin's disease have noncaseating hepatic granulomas even in the absence of involvement of the liver by neoplastic cells. In many cases, unfortunately, the etiology of hepatic granulomas cannot be determined with certainty.

282. The answer is B (1, 3). *(Ackerman, ed 5. p 530.)* The three basic anatomic features of cirrhosis are degeneration or necrosis of hepatocytes, fibrosis, and nodular hepatic regeneration. Fatty change may be seen in alcoholic cirrhosis, but it is not an essential feature of cirrhosis of other etiologies. Bile duct proliferation may occur in cirrhosis secondary to extrahepatic biliary obstruction, but is not an essential feature of cirrhosis in general. Nodules of regenerating hepatocytes may be differentiated from normal hepatic lobules by the absence of a central vein.

283. The answer is C (2, 4). *(Robbins, 1974. pp 1025-1033.)* Chronic alcohol abuse may lead to Laennec's (micronodular) cirrhosis, and is usually accompanied by fat accumulation. Massive hepatic necrosis from viral hepatitis, or drug or chemical toxicity, leads to a random pattern of scarring and regeneration with broad scars and large 3-4 cm nodules.

284-286. The answers are: 284-A, 285-B, 286-B. *(Ackerman, ed 5. p 378. Anderson, ed 6. p 1152.)* Hyperplastic (adenomatous) polyps comprise 80 to 90 percent of all gastric polyps. There is rarely evidence of atypia or malignant transformation in hyperplastic polyps, while malignant changes are noted in from 25 to 72 percent of papillary (villous) adenomas. Hyperplastic polyps of the stomach are generally less than 2 cm while papillary adenomas usually exceed this diameter.

287-290. The answers are: 287-B, 288-C, 289-A, 290-D. *(Anderson, ed 6. pp 1197-1205, 1210-1212.)* Alcohol abuse, alcoholic hepatitis, and Laennec's micronodular cirrhosis are closely related. Although atypical bile duct proliferation is a diagnostic feature of primary biliary cirrhosis, it also occurs in Laennec's micronodular cirrhosis. High serum cholesterol resulting in dermal xanthomas and ulcerative colitis are associated with primary biliary cirrhosis. Laennec's cirrhosis occurs more frequently in men, and primary biliary cirrhosis occurs much more frequently in women (9:1 ratio).

Endocrine System

291. The answer is B. *(Wintrobe, ed 7. p 498.)* Cushing's syndrome may be the result of bilateral adrenal hyperplasia, adrenal neoplasia, or excessive use of ACTH or glucocorticoids. However, bilateral adrenal hyperplasia is the most common etiologic factor found.

292. The answer is A. *(Anderson, ed 6. p 1454.)* Calcifications about the smaller vessels of the brain, especially those of the basal ganglia, are commonly found in hypoparathyroidism and are often visible in skull roentgenograms. The calcifications do not regress with therapy. These lesions are not associated with hypocalcemia from any other cause.

293. The answer is A. *(Anderson, ed 6. p 1088. Beeson, ed 13. p 1879.)* The triad of cystic bone lesions, precocious puberty, and patchy brownish skin pigmentation occurring in young girls is known as Albright's syndrome. The bone lesions are those of fibrous dysplasia, which apparently result from abnormal activity by the bone-forming mesenchyma. Packing of the medullary cavity by fibrous tissue that contains trabeculae of poorly mineralized fibrous bone is seen in the lesions. Recent reports have described cases of fibrous dysplasia in both males and females who have also had a wide variety of endocrine abnormalities, including hyperthyroidism, acromegaly, and Cushing's syndrome.

294. The answer is E. *(Robbins, 1974. p 265.)* Hyalinization and fibrosis of the islets of Langerhans are frequently seen in diabetes mellitus. However, the islets have only subtle defects, such as the loss of beta cells without significant loss of islet cell mass, in up to one-third of the cases of maturity-onset diabetes. Some juvenile diabetic patients have a leukocytic infiltrate in their islets early in the course of the disease.

295. The answer is B. *(Robbins, 1974. p 1323.)* Thyroid hyperfunction is most commonly caused by diffuse primary hyperplasia; less frequently by a hyperfunctioning focus within an adenomatous goiter or a tumor; and only rarely by Hashimoto's thyroiditis.

296. The answer is B. *(Robbins, 1974. p 1311.)* Patients with adrenal insufficiency secondary to pituitary dysfunction do not have the increased melanin pigmentation of the skin and mucous membranes characteristic of primary Addison's disease.

297. The answer is B. *(Anderson, ed 6. p 1433.)* The histologic appearance of colloid storage goiter generally includes abnormally large colloid-filled follicles compressing the intervening small or normal-sized follicles that contain very little colloid. The epithelium of the follicles is predominantly flat cuboidal with occasional epithelial papillary structures protruding into the follicles. In primary hyperplasia with Graves' disease, the follicular epithelium is tall with papillary infoldings and peripheral vacuolation of the colloid. Riedel's struma appears as a marked fibrous tissue replacement of the normal thyroid histology. In Hashimoto's thyroiditis only remnants of thyroid follicles and epithelial cells are found in sheets of lymphocytes with germinal centers.

298. The answer is B. *(Robbins, 1974. pp 1360-1363.)* Craniopharyngiomas are the second most common hypophyseal tumor. They are frequently cystic and calcified. The tumors resemble the embryonic tooth bud or enamel organ, and are also called adamantinomas or ameloblastomas.

299. The answer is B. *(Robbins, 1974. pp 1358-1359.)* Sheehan's syndrome originally consisted of pituitary necrosis secondary to postpartum hemorrhage, but similar changes occur in nonpregnant females and in males. The pituitary damage is thought to result from vascular insufficiency or thrombosis caused by a sudden drop in blood pressure. In the past, symptomatic pituitary necrosis occurred in one-half of all women with severe postpartum hemorrhage.

300. The answer is A. *(Robbins, 1974. p 1351.)* Chronic hypocalcemia, whatever its origin, leads eventually to secondary hyperparathyroidism. Chronic renal failure is the most important cause, but it may also occur in malabsorption, rickets, disseminated metastatic carcinoma, and multiple myeloma.

301. The answer is C. *(Robbins, 1974. p 1343.)* Medullary carcinomas of the thyroid are thought to arise from calcitonin-secreting parafollicular cells. They may be associated with pheochromocytoma, Marfan's syndrome, or neurofibromas. These carcinomas do not take up iodine, and are not dependent on the pituitary.

302. The answer is B. *(Robbins, 1974. pp 1311-1313.)* Adrenal hemorrhage and necrosis secondary to overwhelming meningococcal infection and bacteremia is known as Waterhouse-Friderichsen syndrome. It usually affects children, and is characterized by cutaneous petechiae, followed by circulatory collapse and death within 24 hours. Prompt diagnosis and treatment with steroids and antibiotics may allow recovery.

303. The answer is C. *(Robbins, 1974. pp 1316-1319.)* Pheochromocytoma is a tumor that arises from pheochromocytes, cells that secrete norepinephrine or epinephrine. These tumors are important because they cause a rare but curable form of hypertension. Administration of histamine has been used as a diagnostic test for the presence of a pheochromocytoma, but it causes a high morbidity.

304. The answer is C. *(Robbins, 1974. p 1365.)* Hypersecretion of growth hormone causes acromegaly in adults and gigantism in children. An acidophilic adenoma of the pituitary is found in 90 percent of these cases. Ten percent of patients have chromophobe adenomas, and rarely the only abnormality is a microscopic focus of acidophilic hyperplasia.

305. The answer is B. *(Robbins, 1974. p 1369.)* Seventy-five percent of patients with myasthenia gravis have abnormal thymuses. One-third of these patients have thymomas, and the remainder have follicular hyperplasia. The relationship between the thymic abnormality and the muscle weakness has not yet been elucidated. Many patients with myasthenia and thymoma have antibodies reactive with the thymus and with muscle, but so do some patients with thymoma without muscle weakness.

306. The answer is C. *(Robbins, 1974. p 1305.)* Cushing's syndrome is characterized biochemically by excess production of glucocorticoids. Affected patients can have central obesity, moon face, buffalo hump, diabetes mellitus, osteoporosis, hypertension, plethora, hirsutism, amenorrhea, acne, weakness, and emotional lability. There are three general categories of Cushing's syndrome: caused by cortisol-secreting adrenal neoplasms; by ACTH-secreting pituitary tumors; and by ACTH-secreting nonpituitary neoplasms.

307. The answer is E (all). *(Robbins, 1974. p 268.)* Nodular glomerulosclerosis (Kimmelstiel-Wilson disease) and glycogen nephrosis (Armanni-Ebstein lesion) are virtually pathognomonic of diabetes mellitus. Hyaline arteriolosclerosis and diffuse glomerulosclerosis may also be seen in nondiabetics, but are more common in diabetics. Necrotizing papillitis also occurs in nondiabetics, but only in the presence or urinary obstruction or analgesic abuse.

308. The answer is E (all). *(Robbins, 1974. p 1311.)* At one time, bilateral adrenal tuberculosis was the most common cause of Addison's disease, and it still accounts for five to ten percent of cases. Massive bilateral adrenal metastases, as from bronchogenic carcinoma, may rarely cause adrenal insufficiency. Acute adrenal insufficiency is most often caused by necrotizing adrenal hemorrhage.

309. The answer is E. *(Lichtenstein, ed 2. p 107.)* Osteitis fibrosa cystica generalisata is a bone disease which occurs in association with hyperparathyroidism and is usually evidenced by loss of the lamina dura about the teeth, subcortical bone resorption, the presence of "cysts," "brown tumors," epulides, and erosion of distal clavicles.

310-313. The answers are: 310-A, 311-A, 312-B, 313-C. *(Robbins, 1974. p 126.)* Cancers may produce hormones not produced by their normal cells of origin. For example, retroperitoneal fibrosarcomas may produce insulin and lung cancers may produce ACTH. Endocrine neoplasms may produce excess amounts of their normal hormonal products, such as a functioning islet cell adenoma. Renal cell carcinomas may produce erythropoietin.

314-317. The answers are: 314-C, 315-A, 316-B, 317-D. *(Ackerman, ed 5. pp 326-335.)* Both malignant thyroid tumors mentioned, in large series, metastasize most often to lymph nodes. The medullary carcinoma does metastasize more frequently, however, than the papillary carcinoma. Psammoma bodies or calcospherules are present in approximately 40 percent of tumors of the papillary type. They are virtually never seen in medullary carcinoma. Medullary carcinoma associated with hormone-forming tumors is part of Sipple's syndrome, a type of multiple endocrine adenomatosis syndrome. It is associated with pheochromocytomas which are often bilateral, and with parathyroid adenomata. There have been only sporadic reports of associations between thyroid lesions other than medullary carcinoma and hormone-forming tumors. Although medullary carcinomas are more aggressive than papillary carcinomas, neither is a high grade malignancy with poor prognosis. The undifferentiated carcinomas of the thyroid gland of large, small, and spindle cell type closely fit the description mentioned in the question.

Genitourinary System

318. The answer is C. *(Robbins, 1974. pp 1143-1144.)* Wilms' tumor is the second most common visceral tumor of children under the age of 10 years. The tumors probably arise from the primitive renal blastema, and may contain a variety of cell and tissue components of mesodermal origin. They are usually unilateral and may grow to huge size.

319. The answer is A. *(Stanbury, ed 3. p 196.)* Primary hyperoxaluria results in overproduction of oxalic acid and consequent precipitation of insoluble calcium oxalate salt in the renal parenchyma. The resulting nephrolithiasis and nephrocalcinosis lead to chronic renal failure and early death from uremia.

320. The answer is D. *(Beeson, ed 13. p 1193.)* Renal vein thrombosis may occur as a result of its invasion by hypernephroma, or compression by malignant metastases to retroperitoneal lymph nodes. Other causes include extension from thrombophlebitis of the legs, dehydration, and congestive heart failure. The most common underlying renal disease is, however, renal amyloidosis.

321. The answer is C. *(Robbins, 1974. p 1092.)* Circulating antibodies reactive with the glomerular basement membrane in Goodpasture's syndrome will bind in a linear pattern along the entire length of the glomerular basement membrane which is their specific antigen.

322. The answer is D. *(Ackerman, ed 5. p 634.)* In a patient with a surgically correctable lesion of the renal artery, the corresponding kidney, which is potentially the least damaged one, should be saved. The contralateral kidney may be severely affected with arteriolonephrosclerosis and could perpetuate the hypertension if not removed. In a patient with parenchymal renal disease leading to hypertension, such as pyelonephritis, removal of the affected kidney may relieve the hypertension.

323. The answer is D. *(Robbins, 1974. pp 1090-1106.)* The basement membrane thickening in systemic lupus erythematosus and membranous glomerulonephritis is thought to result from deposition of immune complexes. The pathogenesis of this same lesion in diabetes mellitus and renal vein thrombosis is unknown.

324. The answer is C. *(Ackerman, ed 5. p 625.)* It may be difficult to distinguish grossly between chronic glomerulonephritis and chronic pyelonephritis. However, chronic glomerulonephritis involves both kidneys typically, and does not cause deformation of the pelvis and calyces. Microscopically, virtually all glomeruli are affected in chronic glomerulonephritis, while in pyelonephritis the changes may be patchy. Inflammation of the pelvis also may be recognized microscopically in chronic pyelonephritis.

325. The answer is B. *(Robbins, 1974. p 1161.)* All bladder cancers classically produce painless hematuria. The prognosis depends on the histologic pattern, the grade of anaplasia, and the clinical stage. Transitional cell tumors are the most common and range from well differentiated, relatively benign papillomas to anaplastic, highly aggressive tumors.

326. The answer is E. *(Robbins, 1974. p 1195.)* Carcinoma of the prostate is the most common malignancy in adult males. It exists in two forms: a common, small localized lesion that is an incidental finding in up to 46 percent of men over 50-years-old at autopsy; and the less common but clinically significant form that may metastasize and kill. It is not known whether the localized form progresses to the more aggressive form if untreated.

327. The answer is B. *(Davis, ed 2. p 721.)* Glomerulonephritis may be seen following infection with types 4, 12, 18, 25, and other types, but is usually associated with infection by type 12, group A streptococci. Rheumatic fever following streptococcal infection is associated with group A organisms of various types.

328. The answer is D. *(Robbins, 1974. p 1239.)* Tuberculous salpingitis is almost invariably a secondary complication of tuberculosis elsewhere in the body. The fallopian tubes are probably seeded hematogenously, and then the process spreads to other genital organs, such as the endometrium. Tuberculous salpingitis is extremely rare at present.

329. The answer is B. *(Robbins, 1974. p 1257.)* Ectopic pregnancy refers to implantation of the fetus in any site other than the normal uterine location. The most common site is within the tubular portion of the fallopian tubes, but other sites, including the ovary, abdominal cavity, and the intrauterine portion of the fallopian tube, may be involved. Any delay or obstruction in the passage of the ovum may lead to ectopic implantation. The most important cause is chronic inflammatory disease within the tubes.

330. The answer is A. *(Robbins, 1974. p 1224.)* The presence of endometrial glands and stroma deep within the myometrium constitutes adenomyosis. These glands often have been demonstrated to be connected to the endometrial mucosa, by serial sectioning. The glands in adenomyosis are derived from the basal layer of the endometrium, and are therefore unresponsive to hormones.

331. The answer is C. *(Robbins, 1974. pp 1223-1224.)* Plasma cells are seen in the late stages of primary chronic endometritis and in the secondary forms of endometritis. Neutrophils, lymphocytes, histiocytes, and eosinophils may be present during the normal menstrual cycle. Only the plasma cell cannot be considered a normal inhabitant of the endometrium. Chronic endometritis of the secondary form occurs in women with pelvic inflammatory disease, tuberculous salpingitis, or puerperal infections.

332. The answer is C. *(Robbins, 1974. p 1217.)* Carcinoma of the cervix is associated with chronic cervicitis, early and frequent intercourse, and uncircumsized sexual partners. It may be preceded by carcinoma in situ. The administration of diethylstilbestrol to pregnant women induced an increased frequency of vaginal adenocarcinoma in the exposed offspring, but a relationship between estrogen and carcinoma of the cervix has not been shown.

333. The answer is A. *(Anderson, ed 6. pp 1544, 1547, 1551-1553.)* Adenofibromas, entodermal sinus tumors, and serous cystadenomas are diffusely cystic. Brenner tumors are focally cystic. Hilar cell tumors are solid masses.

334. The answer is B. *(Ackerman, ed 5. p 845.)* Mucinous cystadenomas of the ovary may occasionally contain intestinal mucosa and enzymes, suggesting that at least some of the cystadenomas arise from teratomas. The mucinous glands secrete true mucins (acid mucopolysaccharides) and not "pseudomucins."

335. The answer is D. *(Anderson, ed 8. p 40.)* Benign cystic teratomas constitute about 10 percent of cystic ovarian tumors. The cysts contain greasy sebaceous material mixed with a variable amount of hair. The cysts' walls contain skin and skin appendages, including sebaceous glands and hair follicles. A variety of other tissues such as cartilage, bone, tooth, thyroid, respiratory tract epithelium, and intestinal tissue may be found. The presence of skin and skin appendages gives the tumor its other name, "dermoid" cyst. Dermoid cysts are benign, but in two percent one element may become malignant, most frequently the squamous epithelium.

336. The answer is C. *(Ackerman, ed 5. pp 840-846.)* Ovarian cystadenomas are common neoplasms that are often bilateral (15-40 percent) and are frequently papillary. The less malignant lesions tend to be more papillary.

337. The answer is A. *(Ackerman, ed 5. pp 871-872.)* The eponym Krukenberg's tumor designates a bilateral ovarian neoplasm, almost always metastatic from cancer of the gastrointestinal tract, particularly the stomach. It is characterized microscopically by a diffuse infiltration of signet-ring cells containing abundant mucin and by areas of mucoid degeneration.

338. The answer is D. *(Ackerman, ed 5. p 719.)* The presence of hypoplastic and atrophic seminiferous tubules indicates that the patient is probably infertile. However, 25 to 50 percent of patients with a total lack of spermatozoa (azoospermia) may still have a normal testicular biopsy; this usually is diagnostic of bilateral obstruction or the absence of some part of the duct system. Surgical reconstruction may frequently be helpful.

339. The answer is E. *(Robbins, 1974. p 1183.)* Germ cell tumors are the most common neoplasm in 25 to 35-year-old men, and have an overall incidence of 3 per 100,000 male population. The tumors can arise at any age, but the peak incidence occurs between 25 and 35 years and a smaller peak occurs in elderly males. Approximately 97 percent of testicular tumors arise from germ cells. The tumors cause testicular enlargement, are highly malignant, and often have metastasized by the time of clinical presentation.

340. The answer is B. *(Robbins, 1974. pp 1185-1189.)* Seminoma is a malignant germ cell neoplasm and is the most common testicular tumor. In spite of its malignancy and frequent pattern of metastases to lymph nodes in the pelvis and abdomen the prognosis is often good because of susceptibility to radiation therapy. Teratoma, by definition, is the benign counterpart of teratocarcinoma. Leydig cell tumor is synonymous with interstitial cell tumor. These tumors are rare, representing one percent or less of all testicular tumors, and are generally benign. Their significance lies in their ability to produce androgenic hormones. Adenomatoid tumors are benign neoplasms which appear to arise in the epididymis or remnants of müllerian duct tissue.

341. The answer is B. *(Robbins, 1974. p 1196.)* In nearly 75 percent of cases, carcinoma of the prostate arises within the posterior lobe of the gland, almost always in a subcapsular location. In its early phase, this location may make diagnosis by usual means, including needle biopsy, difficult. Benign nodular hyperplasia of the prostate is, however, most often confined to the inner regions of the gland. Sufficient enlargement to cause decreased patency of the urethral lumen or to interfere with the internal sphincter must occur before the classic micturition disturbances become manifest.

342. The answer is A (1, 2, 3). *(Robbins, 1974. p 1120.)* Necrotizing papillitis, also called renal papillary necrosis, results from ischemic necrosis of the renal papillae and adjacent portions of the renal medulla. The lesion is most often, though not invariably, associated with acute and chronic pyelonephritis. Half the cases of necrotizing papillitis have been associated with diabetes, but it is also common in patients who consume large quantities of analgesics containing phenacetin. As seen in sickle cell anemia, it may have a vascular basis.

343. The answer is C (2, 4). *(Robbins, 1974. pp 1117-1122.)* Acute pyelonephritis is a suppurative bacterial infection of the renal tubules, interstitium, and pelvis, usually caused by *E. coli* or other gram-negative organisms. It often follows urinary tract obstruction or instrumentation.

344. The answer is B (1, 3). *(Robbins, 1974. pp 1093-1096.)* Acute poststreptococcal glomerulonephritis usually affects children 5 to 30 days after a streptococcal infection. It is associated with decreased serum complement and increased ASO titer. Ninety-five percent of affected patients recover without sequellae.

345. The answer is B (1, 3). *(Robbins, 1974. pp 1102-1103.)* The nephrotic syndrome is characterized by proteinuria, hypoalbuminemia, generalized edema, and hyperlipidemia. It occurs in a variety of renal diseases including membranous glomerulonephritis and renal vein thrombosis.

346. The answer is E (all). *(Ackerman, ed 5. p 633.)* Many pathologic processes affecting the kidney can lead to hypertension. The three main categories are: renovascular; renal parenchymal; and urinary tract obstruction. The renin-angiotensin system has been implicated in renovascular hypertension, but has not been proven to be of etiologic importance in the latter two categories. The most common parenchymal diseases leading to hypertension are pyelonephritis and hydronephrosis.

347. The answer is C (2, 4). *(Robbins, 1974. pp 284, 349.)* The kidneys are small and scarred in chronic glomerulonephritis and arteriolar nephrosclerosis. They may be pale and slightly swollen in acute tubular necrosis secondary to shock. The kidneys in amyloidosis are usually normal or slightly enlarged.

348. The answer is D (4). *(Anderson, ed 6. p 1111. Strauss, ed 2. pp 1373-1374.)* Lupus erythematosus is virtually unknown in very young children. Acute poststreptococcal glomerulonephritis occurs in an older pediatric population, is a proliferative lesion pathologically, and is not usually associated with hemolytic anemia or fibrin deposition. Lipoid nephrosis shows no glomerular changes with light microscopy. The pathologic picture presented is that of the hemolytic uremic syndrome.

349. The answer is A (1, 2, 3). *(Strauss, ed 2. p 1374.)* Steroids and anticoagulation therapy have produced equivocal results at best. The other statements given are true.

350. The answer is D (4). *(Strauss, ed 2. p 393.)* Ultrastructural studies reveal deposition of fibrin in the mesangium of the glomerulus in addition to deposition of IgG and $\beta_1 C$ globulin in anaphylactoid nephritis.

351. The answer is E (all). *(Anderson, ed 6. pp 782-783, 791-793, 803-804, 1701-1702.)* Scarring is the end-stage glomerular lesion that results from a variety of injuries of infectious, immunologic, and vascular types. When fibrosis reaches this degree, the nature of the original lesion is often obscured.

352. The answer is A (1, 2, 3). *(Robbins, 1974. p 1087.)* Type I polycystic kidney disease is characterized by dilatation and hyperplasia of all renal collecting tubules in an affected individual. The resultant sponge-like kidneys are uniform and bilaterally symmetrical. Bile ducts may also be cystic in affected infants. Type I polycystic kidneys are incompatible with extended life and are therefore found only in infants.

353. The answer is B (1, 3). *(Robbins, 1974. pp 1140-1143.)* The renal cell carcinoma shown has been called a hypernephroma because of its yellow color, which makes it resemble adrenal tissue, and its predilection for arising from the upper pole of the kidney.

354. The answer is E (all). *(Ackerman, ed 5. p 663.)* Renal cell carcinomas may be associated with various systemic manifestations including fever, hepatosplenomegaly, and hepatic dysfunction. They may produce a parathormone-like substance which causes hypercalcemia, or polycythemia secondary to the secretion of an erythropoietin-like substance. The clear cytoplasm contains fat and glycogen.

355. The answer is C (2, 4). *(Robbins, 1974. p 1195.)* Carcinoma of the prostate typically arises in the posterior lobe. Invasion of the capsule, blood vessels, and perineural spaces are helpful diagnostic signs. Metastatic carcinoma usually causes an elevation of the serum acid phosphatase level, but it is not known whether the elevation is due to the greater amount of neoplastic tissue present or to the more ready absorption of the enzyme into the blood stream from the bony metastases. Tumor growth is not estrogen dependent, but may be inhibited by estrogen administration.

356. **The answer is E (all).** *(Robbins, 1974. pp 1159-1165.)* Papillary carcinoma of the bladder usually contains transitional epithelium, but squamous carcinoma and adenocarcinoma may also occur. Papillary carcinoma usually causes hematuria, recurs frequently, and may be related to industrial carcinogens, tobacco tars, metabolites of tryptophan, and mechanical irritation (including parasites).

357. **The answer is B (1, 3).** *(Robbins, 1974. pp 1213-1214.)* Sarcoma botryoides is composed of all the various mesodermal cell types and usually has an extremely poor prognosis, especially in adults.

358. **The answer is A (1, 2, 3).** *(Anderson, ed 6. p 1562.)* Villous swelling occurs focally in any region of the placenta deprived of functional fetal circulation and is not only found in hydatidiform moles. A diagnostic criterion for choriocarcinoma is the absence of villi.

359. **The answer is B (1, 3).** *(Anderson, ed 6. pp 1562-1563.)* A vast majority of hydatidiform moles do not deeply invade the myometrium and occur as a result of fetal death with disappearance of fetal tissue during the first trimester of pregnancy.

360. **The answer is D (4).** *(Hughes, 1968. p 69.)* The vaginal epithelium responds to hormonal stimuli in three ways: by proliferation; maturation; and exfoliation. During the proliferative phase of the menstrual cycle, superficial squamous cells with pyknotic nuclei predominate. During the secretory phase, numerous intermediate cells with vesicular nuclei are seen. An atrophic postmenopausal vaginal smear will contain few, if any, well-differentiated mature squamous cells, reflecting the lack of estrogen stimulation.

361. **The answer is C (2, 4).** *(Robbins, 1974. pp 1224-1227.)* Endometriosis consists of endometrial glands and stroma present in the myometrium (adenomyosis) or other pelvic organs (endometriosis externa). Extrauterine endometriosis can be particularly responsive to ovarian hormones and can produce periodic bleeding. The aberrant endometrium in adenomyosis, however, is usually derived from the nonfunctional stratum basale and these foci rarely bleed during menses.

362. **The answer is A (1, 2, 3).** *(Robbins, 1974. p 1228.)* Cystic endometrial hyperplasia refers to the abnormal growth of endometrium associated with either an absolute or relative estrogen excess. It is a common finding at the time of menopause and in conditions causing an absolute excess of estrogen, i.e., Stein-Leventhal syndrome, functioning granulosa and thecal cell ovarian tumors, or the exogenous administration of estrogenic substances. The microscopic findings in an endometrial biopsy are dominated by the marked dilatation of the endometrial glands giving the tissue section the appearance of Swiss cheese. The glands are lined by benign columnar epithelium which is nonsecretory.

363. The answer is A (1, 2, 3). *(Robbins, 1974. pp 1206, 1238-1239.)* Salpingitis from infection with gonococci or other organisms may cause a tubo-ovarian abscess. Resolution with scarring of the tubes can cause sterility. The primary lesion of syphilis is the chancre, which usually occurs on the vulva.

364. The answer is B (1, 3). *(Robbins, 1974. p 1213.)* Female children exposed to diethylstilbestrol (DES) in utero have a greatly increased risk of developing vaginal adenocarcinoma. Vaginal adenosis may be found in the absence of diethylstilbestrol exposure, but is present in virtually all females exposed to DES in utero. The adenocarcinoma which develops in the areas of vaginal adenosis may resemble endocervical, endometrial, or tubal carcinoma.

365. The answer is B (1, 3). *(Robbins, 1974. p 1261.)* Choriocarcinomas occur with the following incidence: 50 percent arise in moles; 25 percent follow abortions; approximately 22 percent arise in normal pregnancies; and the remainder arise in ectopic pregnancies and genital and extragenital teratomas. They also occur in teratomas in males. A cure rate of up to 80 percent may be obtained with chemotherapy.

366. The answer is E (all). *(Robbins, 1974. p 1235.)* Endometrial carcinoma tends to occur in middle-age to elderly women and has a peak incidence in the sixth decade. It is more prevalent in nulliparous women and women with hypertension, obesity, diabetes mellitus, thyroid abnormalities, and breast carcinoma than in the normal population. These associations may be related in some undetermined manner to hormone disturbances, though a definite link has not been proven.

367. The answer is C (2, 4). *(Robbins, 1974. pp 1232-1235.)* Leiomyomas (fibroids) are benign smooth muscle tumors which are the most common tumors in women. They may proliferate and enlarge during pregnancy, and become necrotic and calcified postmenopausally.

368. The answer is D (4). *(Anderson, ed 6. pp 1543, 1547, 1552-1553.)* Serous cystadenoma is epithelial in origin, thecoma is stromal in origin, and the Brenner tumor is dimorphic, consisting of stromal and epithelial elements. Dysgerminoma is of germ cell origin.

369. The answer is E (all). *(Ackerman, ed 5. pp 865-866.)* The signs of hyperestrogenism produced by ovarian neoplasms such as the granulosa cell tumor or a thecoma are most obvious clinically as precocious puberty in a child or menstrual abnormalities and endometrial hyperplasia in a postmenopausal woman. These tumors may produce uterine enlargement on the basis of muscle hypertrophy and marked endometrial hyperplasia.

370. The answer is D (4). *(Ackerman, ed 5. p 865.)* Meigs' syndrome is a benign ovarian fibroma associated with ascites and occasionally with pleural effusion, usually right-sided. After removal of the fibroma, the ascites and pleural effusion will normally disappear. Since the pleural space does not contain neoplastic cells in Meigs' syndrome, intrapleural administration of chemotherapeutic agents is not required therapy.

371. The answer is A (1, 2, 3). *(Robbins, 1974. pp 1176-1177.)* Bowen's disease is considered by some to be synonymous with carcinoma in situ. Five to ten percent of patients with Queyrat's erythroplasia develop squamous cell carcinoma. Leukoplakia is also considered premalignant and is thought to arise from chronic irritation. Phimosis is simply a congenital or postinflammatory narrowing of the orifice of the prepuce.

372. The answer is A (1, 2, 3). *(Robbins, 1974. p 1198.)* Hematuria is an uncommon finding in patients with prostatic carcinoma, and occurs only with invasion of the mucosa of the bladder or urethra. Metastases to the skeletal system are osteoblastic in nearly 90 percent of cases since this carcinoma stimulates bone formation. Normal prostatic tissue elaborates acid phosphatase and in 50 to 75 percent of patients with carcinoma that has extended beyond the prostatic capsule, the serum acid phosphatase will show significant elevation. Elevation of the serum alkaline phosphatase indicates widespread bone involvement with increased osteoblastic activity.

373. The answer is D (4). *(Robbins, 1974. p 1181.)* Mumps orchitis is rare before puberty. Testicular involvement is most often unilateral, but may be bilateral. The onset is commonly between the fifth and tenth day of illness, as the parotid swelling is subsiding. Some degree of atrophy, caused by pressure necrosis, occurs in about one-third to one-half of the cases of orchitis. The involvement of the testis is, however, usually spotty and seldom results in sterility.

374-378. The answers are: 374-E, 375-B, 376-C, 377-A, 378-D. *(Robbins, 1974. pp 1080-1081. Strauss, ed 2. pp 3-7.)* The ribbonlike basement membrane separates the glomerular capillary lumen, which is lined by endothelial cells, from Bowman's space. Endothelial cells line the capillaries which contain erythrocytes in this electron micrograph. They can be distinguished from epithelial cells by their lack of foot processes. Foot processes come into direct contact with the basement membrane and represent extensions of the epithelial cells lining Bowman's space. In certain diseases, such as lipoid nephrosis, these processes fuse. The capillary lumen is easily distinguished from Bowman's space by the presence of erythrocytes and other cellular blood elements. Bowman's space can be distinguished from the capillary lumen by the adjacent foot processes which are part of the glomerular epithelial cells.

379-381. The answers are: 379-B, 380-A, 381-C. *(Robbins, 1974. pp 1134-1138.)* Uric acid stones may lead to urinary tract obstruction and hydronephrosis. Disseminated intravascular coagulation secondary to a number of causes including shock, toxemia, and septicemia, is thought to be the final common pathway leading to diffuse cortical necrosis. Embolism, resulting from endocarditis or a mural thrombus overlying a myocardial infarct, is the most common cause of focal renal infarction.

382-384. The answers are: 382-A, 383-E, 384-E. *(Robbins, 1974. pp 268, 1120, 1132-1135.)* Renal arteriolar changes in malignant hypertension include hyperplastic arteriolar nephrosclerosis and necrotizing arteriolitis with fibrinoid necrosis. Diabetic patients may develop nodular glomerulosclerosis (Kimmelstiel-Wilson disease). Necrotizing papillitis is a variant of acute pyelonephritis also seen typically in diabetic patients.

385-388. The answers are: 385-C, 386-B, 387-A, 388-D. *(Anderson, ed 6. pp 822, 1319. Strauss, ed 2. pp 1323-1324.)* Although the prognosis for nephroblastoma in infants under the age of one year has improved with combined therapy, like neuroblastoma it still can metastasize widely and kill. Neuroblastomas frequently present with osseous metastases, but nephroblastomas metastasize to bones only rarely. Nephroblastomas differentiate into a variety of mesenchymal structures and embryonal rhabdomyoblasts can occupy large portions of the tumor. Almost all nephroblastomas and neuroblastomas arise in children under the age of five years, although occasional examples are seen in adolescents.

Nervous System

389. The answer is B. *(Robbins, 1974. p 1530.)* Herpes zoster (shingles) produces a vesicular eruption along the distribution of a cranial or spinal sensory nerve. The inflammatory lesions occur in the dorsal root ganglia, in the spinal cord, and, to a varying degree, in the corresponding peripheral nerves. Pain is severe.

390. The answer is C. *(Robbins, 1974. p 1502.)* Toxoplasmosis is caused by an obligate, intracellular, protozoan, *Toxoplasma gondii*. The definitive host is the cat, but other animals such as cattle may be intermediate hosts. In newborns, toxoplasmosis may cause destructive granulomatous inflammations of the leptomeninges, brain, and eye, and can be fatal. In adults, the majority of infections are asymptomatic.

391. The answer is D. *(Wintrobe, ed 7. pp 814-815, 1801-1804.)* Persistent remitting, bulging fontanelles, convulsions, focal neurologic signs, and persistent fever are often indicative of subdural effusion in an infant with *H. influenzae* meningitis. Hemophilus is one of the two common causes of meningitis in childhood and infancy; the other is meningococcus. *Hemophilus* meningitis is characterized by a heavy plastic-like fibrin-rich exudate which collects about the base of the brain and brain stem. Because of the localization, the foramina and aqueducts may be obstructed producing a progressive internal hydrocephalus.

392. The answer is A. *(Robbins, 1974. p 1499.)* Infection of nerve cells by poliovirus leads to swelling and chromatolysis of the cytoplasm, with displacement of the nucleus. Later, cell destruction occurs with breakdown of the nuclear and cytoplasmic membranes. Dead cells are eventually replaced by an astroglial scar. The anterior horn cells of the spinal cord are the most severely affected. The motor nuclei of the cranial nerves may be affected to a lesser degree.

393. The answer is A. *(Stanbury, ed 3. p 615.)* Ganglioside lipidosis or Tay-Sachs disease results in blindness associated with a cherry-red spot in the retina. Affected individuals also demonstrate developmental retardation, paralysis, and dementia. The disease is usually fatal by the age of three to four years.

394. The answer is B. *(Robbins, 1974. p 1505.)* Neurons are the cells in the central nervous system most vulnerable to anoxia. The cells affected earliest are those in Sommer's sector of the hippocampus, followed by the Purkinje cells of the cerebellum. The primary motor areas and receptive areas are relatively spared in contrast to the severe involvement of the association areas.

395. The answer is C. *(Robbins, 1974. p 1535.)* Wernicke's disease is an encephalopathy characterized by mental confusion, nystagmus, extraocular palsies, prostration, and often by death. It occurs commonly in alcoholics, and is a consequence of thiamine deficiency. The most impressive lesions are in the mamillary bodies.

396. The answer is C. *(Robbins, 1974. p 1510.)* Hemorrhage into the brain may be caused by hypertensive cerebral vascular disease, by trauma, by rupture of aneurysms or angiomas, by blood dyscrasias, and by bleeding into tumors. Atherosclerosis in the absence of hypertension is not a cause. Recovery from a hypertensive hemorrhage is very infrequent. Most hypertensive hemorrhages occur in the cerebral hemispheres, especially in the putamen and claustrum. The thalamus is also frequently affected.

397. The answer is C. *(Robbins, 1974. pp 1510-1512.)* Hypertension is the most common cause of intracranial hemorrhage, and 80 percent of hypertensive hemorrhages are in the cerebral hemispheres. True hemorrhage can be distinguished from a hemorrhagic infarct by the fact that the latter corresponds to the area supplied by a given artery, while the former may overlap arterial supplies.

398. The answer is D. *(Ackerman, ed 5. p 1249.)* Schwannomas generally appear as extremely cellular spindle cell neoplasms, sometimes with metaplastic elements of bone, cartilage, and skeletal muscle. Medulloblastomas occur exclusively in the cerebellum and microscopically are highly cellular with uniform nuclei, scant cytoplasm, and in about one-third of cases rosette formation centered by neurofibrillary material. Oligodendrogliomas are marked by foci of calcification in 70 percent of cases. Microscopically, the most common pattern is a uniform cellularity composed of round cells with small dark nuclei, clear cytoplasm, and a clearly defined cell membrane. Ependymomas are distinguished by ependymal rosettes which are duct-like structures with a central lumen around which columnar tumor cells are arranged in a concentric fashion.

399. The answer is B. *(Robbins, 1974. p 1516.)* Astrocytomas are the most common tumors arising from glial cells. They range in malignancy from a low grade, slowly invasive tumor to the highly malignant glioblastoma multiforme. The more malignant lesions are accompanied by hemorrhage, necrosis, capillary proliferation, and the formation of small cysts.

400. The answer is A. *(Robbins, 1974. p 1521.)* Medulloblastoma, more than any other glioma, has a tendency to seed through the subarachnoid space to involve brain and spinal cord. Midline medulloblastomas expand into the fourth ventricle and produce ventricular obstructive symptoms. The other tumors listed may disseminate through the cerebrospinal pathways but do so less commonly than the medulloblastoma.

401. The answer is E. *(Robbins, 1974. pp 1520-1521.)* Medulloblastomas always arise in the cerebellum, and two-thirds of them occur in children. They are thought to arise from the external granular layer of the cerebellar folia. The tumors are initially highly radiosensitive, but total recovery is very rare.

402. The answer is E. *(Anderson, ed 8. pp 984, 998-1000.)* Neuroblastoma is a tumor of the sympathetic neuroblast and is of neuronal, and not glial, origin. Neurofibromas are formed as a result of the proliferation of all peripheral nerve elements: neurites, Schwann cells, fibroblasts, and probably perineural cells. Neurilemomas originate from Schwann cells and are encapsulated. The malignant schwannoma is also referred to as neurogenic sarcoma, or neurofibrosarcoma. It is the malignant counterpart of neurofibroma. Neuromas most often follow trauma and are, therefore, commonly referred to as traumatic neuromas. They contain all the peripheral nerve elements.

403. The answer is B. *(Robbins, 1974. p 1543.)* Motor neuron disease is a progressive disorder of the motor neurons in the cerebral cortex, brain stem, and spinal cord which occurs in different forms, depending upon the involvement of one or more of these anatomic sites. In progressive muscular atrophy, there is predominant involvement of anterior horn cells with remittent weakness and atrophy of muscles, but no evidence of corticospinal tract dysfunction; in amyotrophic lateral sclerosis there is corticospinal involvement. The basic pathologic process in both is similar.

404. The answer is C. *(Robbins, 1974. pp 1319-1320.)* The neuroblastoma is a highly malignant tumor which occurs most frequently in children and young adolescents. About 50 percent of neuroblastomas are found in the adrenal gland, and most of the remainder occur in association with the sympathetic chain. When these tumors develop in the retina, they are called retinoblastomas. The tumor cells form rosettes with nerve fibrils growing into the center of each rosette.

405. The answer is B (1, 3). *(Robbins, 1974. p 1521.)* Meningiomas are more common in adults than children and occur nearly twice as often in women as in men. The tumors apparently arise from fibroblastic elements normally found in arachnoidal tissue. Because meningiomas occur outside the brain parenchyma and grow slowly, they are uniquely amenable to surgical treatment. Meningiomas are typically discrete and encapsulated so that symptoms occur as the growing tumor displaces and compresses normal brain parenchyma.

406. The answer is E (all). *(Robbins, 1974. pp 1510-1512.)* Hypertensive hemorrhage into the brain is the most common cause of death from a cerebral vascular accident. Infarcts are more common, but are not as frequently fatal as hypertensive hemorrhages. Hemorrhage may also occur secondary to trauma, aneurysm rupture, and bleeding diathesis in a blood dyscrasia.

407. The answer is B (1, 3). *(Robbins, 1974. p 1506.)* The major causes of cerebral infarction are cerebral arteriosclerosis, cerebral arteritis, and cerebral embolism. Emboli to cerebral vessels come chiefly from the heart, either from thrombi formed in the fibrillating left atrium, from mural thrombi overlying a myocardial infarct, or from valvular material in endocarditis. An infarct may either be ischemic or hemorrhagic, depending on whether the blood flow to the infarcted area is eventually restored leading to hemorrhage into the infarct.

408. The answer is A (1, 2, 3). *(Robbins, 1974. p 1510.)* Hypertensive hemorrhages occur nearly 80 percent of the time in the cerebral hemispheres. They affect, in decreasing order, the putamen and claustrum, the thalamus, and the white matter (rare). Approximately 10 percent of hypertensive hemorrhages occur in the pons or midbrain and the remaining 10 percent occur in the cerebellum.

409. The answer is C (2, 4). *(Robbins, 1974. pp 1488-1490.)* The cause of the common hydrocephalus of the antenatal and neonatal period is unclear. Excess production or inadequate resorption of the cerebrospinal fluid may play a role. Stenosis of the aqueduct of Sylvius is not infrequently seen, but stenosis of the foramina of Magendie and Luschka is very rare.

410. The answer is E (all). *(Anderson, ed 6. p 1814.)* Kernicterus is a neurologic complication of severe, unconjugated hyperbilirubinemia, which may develop in a jaundiced newborn. Normally, the binding of unconjugated bilirubin by albumin restricts pigment diffusion into tissue cells. However, when the unconjugated bilirubin concentration exceeds the albumin-binding capacity, the lipid-soluble, unconjugated bilirubin is free to diffuse through the blood-brain barrier. Depression of the plasma albumin level, administration of drugs that bind to albumin displacing bilirubin, and metabolic acidosis all predispose to kernicterus. The bile pigments are noted to discolor the globi pallidi, subthalamic nuclei, hippocampi, dentate nuclei, and inferior olivary nuclei most commonly.

411. The answer is D (4). *(Robbins, 1974. p 1530.)* In multiple neuritis there is partial destruction of some peripheral nerves, and the distribution is usually bilateral. Atrophy and flaccid paralysis are characteristic findings and not fasciculations. The distal portions of the extremities are most severely affected.

412. The answer is C (2, 4). *(Robbins, 1974. p 1542.)* The pathology of Parkinson's disease remains controversial as to the significance of the observed lesions. In the disease there is a reduction of pigment in the substantia nigra, and nerve cell loss and degeneration. Nigral cells may show rounded intracytoplasmic inclusions which are termed Lewy bodies. A small lenticular nucleus and atrophy of the ansa lenticularis have also been observed.

413. The answer is E (all). *(Robbins, 1974. p 1534.)* The term leukoencephalopathies is used to encompass a group of rare diseases of childhood in which the lesions are thought to result from a congenital defect in formation and/or maintenance of myelin. Pelizaeus-Merzbacher disease, Krabbe's disease (globoid cell leukodystrophy), metachromatic leukodystrophy (sulfatide lipidosis), and Schilder's disease (progressive subcortical encephalopathy) all fall under this category.

414. The answer is B (1, 3). *(Robbins, 1974. p 1531.)* Demyelinization occurs in many pathologic processes of the central nervous system, but the demyelinating diseases are those in which loss of myelin without proportionate loss of axis cylinders is the major manifestation. Only three important diseases fall within this strict definition: postinfectious encephalomyelitis; multiple sclerosis; and progressive multifocal leukoencephalopathy. Postinfectious encephalomyelitis can follow measles, chickenpox, smallpox, or inoculation for smallpox or rabies. The etiology of multiple sclerosis is unknown.

415. The answer is E (all). *(Robbins, 1974. p 1531.)* Refsum's disease is characterized by hypertrophic neuropathy, ataxia, progressive nerve deafness, retinitis pigmentosa, and a high cerebrospinal fluid protein count. It is a result of a metabolic disorder in which an exogenous fatty acid, phytanic acid, accumulates in tissues. The ataxia is thought to be due to the combined effects of polyneuritis and a varying degree of central nervous system fiber degeneration. Refsum's disease is also known as heredopathia atactica polyneuritiformis.

416. The answer is A (1, 2, 3). *(Robbins, 1974. p 1496.)* Tabes dorsalis causes bilateral degeneration of dorsal nerve roots and the posterior funiculi. During the early phase of the disease there are sharp attacks of pain because of irritation of the dorsal nerve roots, but later there is a progressive loss of sensitivity to pain, vibration, and proprioceptive stimuli. The interruption of the stretch reflex may result in a positive Romberg sign. The pathogenesis of tabes dorsalis is controversial. Postulates include tabes as a result of focal leptomeningeal inflammation of the dorsal roots, changes in the structure of the dorsal root ganglia, and of a toxic product or metabolic disorder, rather than tissue infestation by *Treponema*.

417. The answer is D (4). *(Robbins, 1974. p 1543.)* Amyotrophic lateral sclerosis is a disease of unknown etiology which may have a prolonged course but is eventually fatal. Destruction of motor neurons occurs in the anterior gray horns, together with bilateral degeneration of the pyramidal tracts, and thus the clinical deficit is mixed upper and lower motor neuron disease. Weakness, atrophy, and fasciculations occur in some muscles, usually in the hands, and spasticity and hyperreflexia in others, usually in the legs. Amyotrophic lateral sclerosis, progressive spinal muscular atrophy, and progressive bulbar palsy differ from one another only in the distribution of the lesions.

418. The answer is A (1, 2, 3). *(Robbins, 1974. p 1544.)* Syringomyelia is a disease in which there is softening and cavitation around the central canal of the spinal cord. The lateral spinothalamic tracts are interrupted as they cross ventral to the canal resulting in loss of pain and temperature sense in a segmental distribution (the long tracts are not disturbed). The cause of syringomyelia remains unknown. At autopsy the spinal cord is found to contain a cyst surrounded by scar tissue and filled with fluid. The overlying leptomeninges are often thickened. The extent of spinal cord degeneration depends on the size of the cyst and the amount of resulting gliosis.

419. The answer is B (1, 3). *(Robbins, 1974. pp 1536-1537.)* Subacute combined degeneration is a disease often seen in association with pernicious anemia or other nutritional disturbances. The posterior funiculi and pyramidal tracts undergo degeneration, but the gray matter is only rarely affected. Motor weakness with spasticity is the characteristic result.

420. The answer is E (all). *(Robbins, 1974. pp 1539-1540.)* Alzheimer's disease is said to be the major cause of organic mental change in elderly patients. If the syndrome of parenchymal lesions of cortical atrophy, neuron loss, neurofibrillar degeneration, and senile plaques occurs earlier in life, the resultant clinical picture is termed presenile dementia by clinicians. Progression usually results in complete dementia.

421. The answer is A (1, 2, 3). *(Ackerman, ed 5. p 1249.)* Glioblastoma multiforme is often observed to have regions of cystic degeneration, hemorrhage, and necrosis. Microscopically, highly cellular areas are interspersed with large foci of necrosis. The tumor cells show a wide diversity of shape and size, i.e., "multiforme." No perinuclear "halos" are generally encountered, but cytoplasmic invaginations within folds of the nuclear membrane may be present and may be mistaken for intranuclear inclusions. The tumors rank high among malignancies with a poor prognosis: the two-year mortality approaches 90 percent. Glioblastomas are unique among primary central nervous system tumors in producing extracranial metastases, commonly to lung and cervical lymph nodes.

422-426. The answers are: 422-B, 423-B, 424-A, 425-C, 426-D. *(Anderson, ed 6. pp 1417-1418, 1833-1846.)* The medulloblastoma (neuroblastoma) is a malignant neuroglial neoplasm occurring most frequently in children during the first decade of life. It is restricted to the cerebellum. The hemangioblastoma is a highly vascular neoplasm, thought to be a form of meningioma (angioblastic). It occurs in all portions of the central nervous system but is most common in the cerebellum. The chromophobe adenoma accounts for approximately two-thirds of all pituitary adenomas and occurs in the anterior lobe of the gland. The glioblastoma multiforme, a highly malignant astrocytoma, is common in adults and occurs most frequently in the cerebral hemispheres. Meningiomas are benign neoplasms that arise in the leptomeninges which cover the brain and spinal cord. They often compress, but rarely invade, brain tissue.

427-433. The answers are: 427-E, 428-E, 429-A, 430-C, 431-B, 432-D, 433-C. *(Robbins, 1974. pp 1479-1545.)* Creutzfeldt-Jakob disease, kuru, and subacute sclerosing panencephalitis (SSPE) are classified as diseases caused by slow viruses with incubation periods measured in years. The distinguishing feature of SSPE is the Cowdry A intranuclear inclusions in the cortical neurons. A measles-like virus has been isolated from the brains of patients with SSPE. Kuru is the disease of the Fore tribe of New Guinea which has been linked to transmission by cannibalism of diseased brains. Krabbe's disease and metachromatic leukodystrophy are leukoencephalopathies thought to result from congenital defects in formation or maintenance of myelin. Multiple sclerosis is also a disease of the white matter but its pathogenesis is not yet known. Amyotrophic lateral sclerosis has as its fundamental pathologic process degeneration of corticospinal or corticobulbar pathways, and degeneration of motor nerve cells of the spinal cord and brain stem.

434-439. The answers are: 434-B, 435-A, 436-C, 437-A, 438-E, 439-D. *(Robbins, 1974. pp 1479-1545.)* Lewy bodies are rounded intracytoplasmic inclusions in the cells of the substantia nigra found in the brains of patients with idiopathic parkinsonism. Postencephalitic parkinsonism represents one of the complications of encephalitis lethargica. Neurofibrillary tangles result from an alteration of the neurofibrillar apparatus so that the fibrils appear thickened and tortuous, forming a tangled skein within the cytoplasm. Neurofibrillary tangles are also seen in Alzheimer's disease. Herpes simplex encephalitis causes necrotizing lesions with type A inclusions in oligodendroglia and occasional neurons. The lesions of Creutzfeldt-Jakob disease are spongiform areas of degeneration of the gray matter particularly in the cerebral cortex. Corpora amylacea are small hyaline-appearing masses of degenerated cells found in a number of tissues; they are not thought to be specific for any known disease.

Skeletomuscular System

440. The answer is A. *(Robbins, 1974. p 1464.)* Metastases account for the majority of bone tumors, followed in frequency by multiple myeloma and osteogenic sarcoma.

441. The answer is C. *(Anderson, ed 6. p 1707. Salter, 1970. p 171.)* The lower thoracic and lumbar vertebrae and their corresponding disks are involved in over 50 percent of cases of tuberculosis of bone and joints.

442. The answer is A. *(Lichtenstein, ed 2. p 52.)* Nutrient arteries to long bones divide to supply the metaphyses and diaphyses. In the metaphyses, the arteries become arterioles and finally form capillary loops adjacent to epiphyseal plates. This anatomic feature allows bacteria to settle in the region of the metaphysis and makes it the site initially involved in hematogenous osteomyelitis. When infected bone undergoes vascular and osteoclastic resorption, it is replaced by fibrous connective tissue. Persistent chronic osteomyelitis is often associated with sequelae which include amyloidosis and the appearance of malignant tumors in old sinus tracts within the damaged bone.

443. The answer is C. *(Wintrobe, ed 7. p 1676.)* Letterer-Siwe disease is primarily a disease of the reticuloendothelial system. It causes localized bone destruction (particularly in the calvaria), purpura, enlargement of the spleen, progressive anemia, and usually results in death. The nature of the underlying defect is not known.

444. The answer is E. *(Beeson, ed 13. p 152. Robbins, 1974. p 1466.)* The most common pattern of joint involvement seen in psoriatic arthritis is a scattered, asymmetrical involvement of the interphalangeal joints of the hands and feet. Much less common, but characteristic of psoriatic arthritis, is the exclusive involvement of distal interphalangeal joints. The joint involvement is often morphologically indistinguishable from the changes of rheumatoid arthritis. The clinical course and features warrant the separation of these entities.

445. The answer is A. *(Lichtenstein, ed 2. p 284.)* The roentgenographic findings in rheumatoid arthritis parallel and reflect the pathologic changes. The earliest radiologic sign is soft tissue swelling. The swelling may be around the proximal interphalangeal joints, metacarpophalangeal joints, or radiocarpal joints. Other early manifestations include thickening of the joint capsule, and significant osteoporosis which is probably not entirely related to steroid therapy. With long-standing arthritis, osteoporosis is a common finding and erosion of bone around the involved joints and narrowing of joint spaces are radiologic findings.

446. The answer is A. *(Anderson, ed 8. p 969.)* Rheumatoid arthritis frequently affects the small joints of the hands and feet. The larger joints are involved later. Subcutaneous nodules, with a necrotic focus surrounded by palisades of proliferating cells, are seen in some cases. In the joints, the synovial membrane is thickened by a granulation tissue pannus which is infiltrated by many inflammatory cells. Nodular collections of lymphocytes resembling follicles are characteristically seen. The thickened synovial membrane may develop villous projections, and the joint cartilage is attacked and destroyed.

447. The answer is B. *(Robbins, 1974. pp 1195-1198.)* Carcinoma of the prostate usually arises in the subcapsular portion of the posterior lobe. Spread occurs principally to the skeletal system, usually affecting the vertebral column first. Skeletal metastases are usually osteoblastic.

448. The answer is D. *(Robbins, 1974. p 1443.)* Osteomalacia is characterized by inadequate mineralization of the bone matrix, resulting in an increase in the relative amount of osteoid tissue. Mineralization may lag behind osteoid synthesis by several weeks, rather than by the normal six to ten days. Osteomalacia may be caused by vitamin D deficiency, hypophosphatemia with normal vitamin D intake, or conditions with normal calcium, phosphorus, and vitamin D, such as fluoride intoxication.

449. The answer is A. *(Robbins, 1974. p 1433.)* Osteogenesis imperfecta is a hereditary trait characterized by defective synthesis of connective tissue, including bone matrix. The skeletal parts are thin and porous, with slender trabeculae. Fractures are common, and deafness may result from involvement of the bones of the middle ear.

450. The answer is A. *(Dahlin, ed 2. p 188.)* Ewing's sarcoma tends to be extensive, sometimes involving the entire shaft of a long bone. It often begins in the diaphyseal marrow and as it grows through the cortex, it may elevate the periosteum in sequential stages. Although the cortex may show only minimal destruction, the periosteal elevation will produce the characteristic multilayering of subperiosteal new bone formation that gives Ewing's tumor a typical "onion skin" appearance in roentgen films.

451. The answer is C. *(Robbins, 1974. pp 1445-1446.)* Paget's disease of bone is characterized by the replacement of normal bone by expanded, soft, poorly mineralized, osteoid tissue. The bones are enlarged, but are soft and easily deformed by the stress of weight-bearing.

452. The answer is A. *(Robbins, 1974. p 1452.)* Osteogenic sarcoma is the leading cause of bone cancer in the young. When it arises after the age of 40, it is usually associated with Paget's disease, prior irradiation, or exposure to radium-containing paints. These lesions usually occur in the long tubular bones, and have a poor prognosis.

453. The answer is A. *(Robbins, 1974. p 1424.)* The inheritance of childhood (Duchenne) muscular dystrophy conforms to an X-linked recessive trait. Muscular dystrophies are genetically determined myopathies characterized by alterations in individual myocytes leading to weakness in the affected muscles. The system of classification is based upon specific patterns of muscle involvement; the pathologic changes in the individual muscle cells are nearly identical in all clinical patterns. The diseased muscle fibers may show an infiltrate of neutrophils, lymphocytes, and macrophages early in the course of the disease. Isolated muscle fiber shrinkage, atrophy, and disappearance of cells is evident later. Finally, widespread muscle cell atrophy, accompanied by an accumulation of fat cells interspersed between remaining muscle fibers, is seen.

454. The answer is B. *(Robbins, 1974. pp 1424-1431.)* Myositis ossificans is a benign condition characterized by fibrous repair of a skeletal muscle tear with secondary cartilage formation, ossification, and calcification. The other lesions mentioned are malignant neoplasms which may contain a variety of mesodermal tissues.

455. The answer is D. *(Robbins, 1974. pp 239-244, 612.)* Hypersensitivity angiitis primarily affects small vessels. Polyarteritis nodosa affects small to medium arteries. In addition to interstitial inflammation (often perivascular), patients with polymyositis have histologic evidence of muscle fiber death. Perivascular inflammation is one of the early skeletal muscle changes in scleroderma (systemic sclerosis). Cystic medial necrosis is not inflammatory, but degenerative.

456. The answer is B. *(Robbins, 1974. pp 1426-1427.)* Seventy-five percent of patients with myasthenia gravis have abnormal thymuses. One-third of the patients have thymomas and the rest have thymic hyperplasia. Many patients have antibodies reactive with skeletal muscle and thymic tissue, and some patients improve following thymectomy. The role of the thymus in the pathogenesis of myasthenia gravis is not, however, understood.

457. The answer is B (1, 3). *(Ackerman, ed 5. p 1040.)* Juxtacortical (parosteal) osteosarcoma is a not too common variant of osteosarcoma. It usually has a less malignant-appearing stroma and may even be confused histologically with a benign condition such as myositis ossificans. It does not follow trauma, and has a better prognosis than osteosarcoma of the shaft or medullary cavity.

458. The answer is A (1, 2, 3). *(Robbins, 1974. pp 1452-1455.)* The characteristic sun-burst appearance shown in the x-ray is due to calcified perpendicular striae within the growing tumor. Osteosarcoma is the most common bone cancer of children and is almost invariably associated with Paget's disease when it occurs in the elderly. The prognosis is extremely poor, with a 5-year survival of 5 to 20 percent.

459. The answer is E (all). *(Edeiken J, Arthritis. JAMA, 232:1366, 1975.)* Calcification of the menisci, or articular cartilages of the knee joints, may be physiologic or pathologic. When physiologic, it is usually asymptomatic. It may occur in chondrocalcinosis, hyperparathyroidism, hemochromatosis, ochronosis, and gout.

460. The answer is B (1, 3). *(Robbins, 1974. pp 1462-1464.)* Metastatic lesions from carcinoma of the prostate are usually osteoblastic. Multiple osteolytic skull lesions are characteristic of multiple myeloma. Myeloma tumors typically produce gelatinous regions of osteolysis within the marrow cavities of involved bones. Coalescence of these foci may cause erosion of the cortical bone and occasionally will produce through-and-through defects. Histologic evidence of bone necrosis with new bone formation is very rare in myeloma lesions, as opposed to in the bone lesions of metastatic prostate carcinoma.

461-465. The answers are: 461-A, 462-B, 463-E, 464-C, 465-D. *(Anderson, ed 6. pp 1727-1744.)* The giant cell tumor of bone usually presents as a lytic lesion involving the epiphyses of long bones. The proximal tibia is a common site. Solitary cysts are loculated, lytic lesions of bone that characteristically abut on the epiphyseal plate in older children and produce cortical irregularities. Regions involved in the benign lesion are prone to fracture. Osteochondromas are cauliflower-like lesions. They contain a core of cortical and medullary bone, and a cartilage cap which decreases in width as age increases. Osteochondromas usually protrude from the metaphyses of long bones and may be multiple. An osteoid-osteoma occurs most frequently in the cortex of the diaphysis of long limb bones particularly the tibia. A small radiolucent nidus is usually surrounded by dense, sclerotic bone. Clinically, the lesion is often associated with pain. Non-ossifying fibroma of bone is usually a well-demarcated, eccentric, lytic metaphyseal lesion most common in the tibia and femur. It is histologically identical to a fibrous cortical defect and consists of a fibroblastic growth without concomitant bone formation.

466-470. The answers are: 466-E, 467-C, 468-D, 469-A, 470-B. *(Williams, ed 5. pp 660-773.)* Osteosarcoma or osteogenic sarcoma is a highly malignant tumor characterized by a fibroblastic sarcomatous stroma in which osteoblastic activity induces the formation of tumor osteoid and new bone. This lesion is not pictured. Primary hyperthyroidism causes increased lacunae size in the trabeculae of the bones associated with increased levels of parathyroid hormone. Rickets can cause a demineralization of the osteoid matrix resulting in areas of decreased mineral density and loss of bone rigidity. Osteoporosis causes enlargement of the spaces of bone (haversian canals) producing a porous appearance. The loss of bony substance results in a brittleness or softness of the bones. Paget's disease is a benign neoplasia of bone characterized by increased skeletal remodeling as indicated by marked increases both in the amount of resorptive activity present and in the amount of bone formation activity.

Skin and Breast

471. The answer is C. *(Robbins, 1974. p 1393.)* Warts may appear on various parts of the body, and have different names depending on their location. For example, the common wart is known as verruca vulgaris, the plantar wart as verruca plantaris, and the venereal wart as condyloma acuminatum. These are all probably variations of the same process. The lesions frequently have intranuclear and cytoplasmic inclusion bodies. They are benign.

472. The answer is E. *(Robbins, 1974. p 1396.)* Seborrheic keratosis has the distinctive feature of appearing to extend above the level of the adjacent epidermis without extending into the dermis. Its superficial location allows the lesion to be removed by scraping without causing much bleeding. The lesions are not premalignant.

473. The answer is C. *(Robbins, 1974. p 1418.)* Urticaria pigmentosa is characterized by the presence of tan to yellow-brown skin papules. The lesions contain mast cells, whose histamine-containing granules may be identified by Giemsa stain, toluidine blue, or periodic acid-Schiff test. The lesions are usually asymptomatic, but may become itchy and form a wheal if rubbed.

474. The answer is D. *(Robbins, 1974. p 1294.)* Cystic hyperplasia ranks ahead of carcinoma as a cause of masses in the breast. Cystic hyperplasia, or fibrocystic disease as it is often termed, is the most important cause of palpable breast abnormalities except in women over 50 years of age. In this group, carcinoma is the most common cause of abnormal breast masses. However, regardless of age group, the clinician must consider all suspicious breast lesions as carcinoma until proven otherwise.

475. The answer is D. *(Robbins, 1974. pp 1272-1276.)* Cystic disease is characterized by hyperplasia of the stroma and ductal epithelium of the breast with subsequent formation of cysts. It rarely forms a solitary mass, but is usually multiple and often bilateral. This is to be expected since the disease is thought to develop from exaggeration of normal breast changes occurring during the menstrual cycle. Thus, the cysts arise from hormonally dilated ducts, rather than obstructed ducts, when phases of epithelial hyperplasia and duct dilatation are not followed by normal regressive changes. This mechanism for the pathogenesis of cystic disease explains why many symptoms are exacerbated during periods of endocrine fluctuation.

476. The answer is B. *(Robbins, 1974. p 1279.)* All the tumors mentioned except lobular carcinoma arise in the mammary duct epithelium, while lobular carcinoma presumably arises from acinar cells. Lobular carcinomas tend to be bilateral far more often than ductal carcinomas, and have a 20 percent chance of occurring in both breasts. They are commonly found to be multicentric in origin within a single breast. Three evolutionary stages are recognized for lobular carcinoma: lobular carcinoma in situ; lobular carcinoma in situ with infiltration; and infiltrative lobular carcinoma without an in situ component. The in situ forms are more prevalent in younger women and are usually found incidentally in mastectomy specimens.

477. The answer is E. *(Robbins, 1974. pp 1279-1288, 1290-1292.)* The first four forms of cancer listed are infiltrating, metastasizing, and inevitably lethal lesions. Cystosarcoma phyllodes is usually a localized lesion, often benign, and when malignant can be cured by operative resection in the majority of cases. Cystosarcoma phyllodes is also called giant fibroadenoma, a more descriptive term for this large tumor which can reach 10-15 cm in diameter. Its bulk alone distorts the breast and may cause pressure necrosis of the overlying skin, giving the impression of an infiltrating necrotic malignancy even when the tumor is histologically benign.

478. The answer is E. *(Anderson, ed 6. pp 1598, 1649-1650.)* In the nipple, an infiltrate of atypical, mucin-positive cells with clear cytoplasm is diagnostic of Paget's disease. It is invariably associated with an underlying cancer of the breast, and usually occurs in middle-aged women.

479. The answer is B. *(Anderson, ed 6. pp 1598, 1649-1650.)* Paget's disease of the nipple is almost invariably associated with an underlying ductal malignancy. Paget's disease arising in the vulva, or other unusual places, is not as frequently associated with deeper cancer.

480. The answer is B. *(Robbins, 1974. p 469.)* Sarcoidosis is a disease of unknown etiology characterized pathologically by epithelioid granulomas without significant necrosis, occurring in any organ or tissue. Lymph nodes are involved in the majority of cases, the group most commonly affected being those in the thorax, principally around the trachea and tracheobronchial bifurcation. Skin lesions are present in about half the cases. The photomicrograph illustrates just such a skin lesion.

481. The answer is A. *(Robbins, 1974. p 1401.)* Most pigmented skin lesions are benign. However, lesions with a suspicious clinical appearance must be biopsied to exclude malignant melanoma. The lesion illustrated is a malignant melanoma, and the prognosis depends in part on the depth of invasion. Lesions which have microscopically reached the subcutaneous fat have a very poor prognosis.

482. The answer is A. *(Anderson, ed 6. pp 466-467.)* As shown, the morphology of the parasite in tissue sections alone is helpful, but not diagnostic for *Onchocerca volvulus*. The nodule's presence in the subcutaneous tissues of the scalp, and the history of travel to Central America where the infestation is endemic, make the diagnosis most likely.

483. The answer is B. *(Robbins, 1974. p 1280.)* The scirrhous carcinoma accounts for three-quarters of all mammary carcinomas and is composed of a dense fibrous stroma containing isolated nests or strands of malignant epithelial cells.

484. The answer is B. *(Robbins, 1974. p 1279.)* Over 90 percent of breast cancers arise in the ductal epithelium. Less than 10 percent arise in lobular structures, such as acini. Sarcomas are very rare in the breasts.

485. The answer is C. *(Robbins, 1974. pp 1270-1276.)* Mammary dysplasia is thought to result from an excessive response to normal hormonal changes. The disease may primarily involve the stroma, the epithelium, or both. Fibrosis, numerous cysts of varying sizes, and extreme ductal proliferation occur. The disease is not inflammatory and should not be called cystic mastitis.

486. The answer is E. *(Robbins, 1974. p 1267.)* Proliferation of neonatal ductal epithelium and periductal connective tissue, caused by maternal hormones, is a common finding in newborns. Abortive secretory activity may even occur. These changes regress by two weeks of age.

487. The answer is D. *(Robbins, 1974. pp 1399, 1409, 1417.)* Keratoacanthoma is a rapidly appearing (and self-regressing) hyperplastic epidermal lesion that mimics squamous cell carcinoma. It is not congenital. Ichthyosis is congenital hypertrophy of the horny layer of the skin. Portwine stains and strawberry hemangiomas are congenital lesions with characteristic increases in the number of dermal capillaries. Both of these lesions are considered to be subtypes of angiomas.

488. The answer is E. *(Robbins, 1974. pp 242, 1382, 1394, 1397, 1415.)* Acanthosis refers to hypertrophy of the prickle-cell layers of the epidermis and is a feature common to all of the lesions mentioned except scleroderma. Scleroderma induces atrophic, rather than hypertrophic skin changes. The sclerotic atrophy of the skin is often accompanied by increased pigmentation as the result of abnormal melanin production in the basal layer of the epidermis. With long-standing disease, even the subcutaneous tissues may undergo sclerotic atrophy.

489. The answer is A (1, 2, 3). *(Robbins, 1974. p 277.)* Excess iron is found in the liver, the pancreas, and many other organs in hemochromatosis. However, it is not known whether the iron deposition is the cause of the tissue damage, or is just a secondary effect. In the pancreas, for example, the severity of the iron deposition bears no relationship to the severity of the diabetes.

490. The answer is A (1, 2, 3). *(Robbins, 1974. p 432.)* Intranuclear inclusions and an intraepithelial location are seen in the vesicular lesions of varicella, variola, and herpes simplex. (The inclusions are only initially confined to the cytoplasm in variola.) Erythematous nodular swellings on the legs and a heavy, perivascular, dermal inflammatory infiltrate are the typical findings in erythema nodosum.

491. The answer is C (2, 4). *(Robbins, 1974. pp 1397-1399, 1414.)* Solar (senile) keratosis and leukoplakia are considered premalignant squamous cell lesions. Solar keratosis, itself, is thought by some pathologists to represent squamous cell carcinoma grade one-half. Twenty to thirty percent of patients with untreated leukoplakia may go on to develop squamous cell carcinomas in these lesions. Seborrheic keratosis is a benign superficial skin tumor commonly found on older individuals. There is no reported premalignant nature in this lesion or in fibroepithelial papilloma which is the common skin tag.

492. The answer is B (1, 3). *(Robbins, 1974. pp 47-48.)* Melanin is a pigment synthesized from tyrosine by melanocytes. Melanocytes are of neuroectodermal origin and give rise to nevi, freckles, and malignant melanomas. They also cause increased skin pigmentation in Addison's disease and in response to sun exposure.

493. The answer is E (all). *(Robbins, 1974. p 1382.)* All of the features mentioned plus edema with clubbing of dermal papillae, and dilatation of straight capillaries in the dermal papillae, are pathognomonic, histologic characteristics of psoriasis. When a lesion is given the diagnosis "psoriasiform dermatitis" this indicates that some but not all of the six characteristics are present. A partial pattern is nondiagnostic, and should not be taken to mean psoriasis, since it is a nonspecific histologic pattern that may be found in other conditions including exfoliative dermatitis, seborrheic dermatitis, chronic contact dermatitis, and neurodermatitis.

494. The answer is D (4). *(Anderson, ed 6. pp 1103, 1106-1108.)* Acinic cell tumors frequently recur and some eventually do metastasize, but many affected patients survive more than ten years. Adenolymphoma (Warthin's tumor) is benign. Squamous cell carcinoma and undifferentiated carcinoma are very malignant lesions with poor five-year survival statistics.

495. The answer is A (1, 2, 3). *(Robbins, 1974. p 1277.)* Familial and genetic factors, as well as prolonged exposure to estrogen, appear to increase the incidence of breast cancer. Breast cancer is, however, more common in nulliparous women than multiparous. Additional groups with an increased incidence of breast cancer (by epidemiologic analysis) include Jewish women, single women, and women in higher socioeconomic classes.

496. The answer is C (2, 4). *(Robbins, 1974. pp 1279, 1288.)* Intraductal papilloma rarely presents as a palpable mass. Most patients with this disease have a nipple discharge which may be bloody, serous, or turbid. Single papillomas vary histologically from benign tumors with normal epithelial cells and no signs of atypia to lesions which are markedly anaplastic with evidence of invasion. Lobular carcinoma in situ does not occur as a palpable lesion, by definition. Only when a lobular carcinoma becomes infiltrative does it become palpable as a mass lesion. Most lobular carcinomas in situ are diagnosed in biopsy or mastectomy specimens which have been removed for other reasons.

497-500. The answers are: 497-E, 498-B, 499-A, 500-D. *(Anderson, ed 6. pp 1615, 1658-1660.)* The halo (Sutton's) nevus is histologically characterized by dermal nevocytic cells surrounded by lymphocytes and zones of depigmentation. Juvenile melanoma is a benign lesion occurring most frequently in the pediatric age group and consisting of spindled, single, and multinucleated giant cells. Approximately 50 percent of adults over the age of 40 years with acanthosis nigricans have an associated visceral malignancy, usually an adenocarcinoma. The blue nevus is a benign, blue-black lesion composed of interlacing fasciculi of spindle cells lying deep in the dermis.

Bibliography

Ackerman, L. V., and Rosai, J. *Surgical Pathology.* 5th ed. St. Louis: C. V. Mosby Co., 1974.

Anderson, W. A., ed. *Pathology.* 6th rev. ed. 2 vols. St. Louis: C. V. Mosby Co., 1971.

Anderson, W. A., and Scotti, T. M. *Synopsis of Pathology.* 8th ed. St. Louis: C. V. Mosby Co., 1972.

Beeson, P. B., and McDermott, W., eds. *Cecil-Loeb Textbook of Medicine.* 13th ed. Philadelphia: Columbia Broadcasting System, W. B. Saunders Co., 1971.

Dahlin, D. C. *Bone Tumors: General Aspects & Data on 3987 Cases.* 2nd ed. Springfield: Charles C. Thomas Publications, 1973.

Davidshohn, I., and Henry, J. B., eds. *Todd-Sanford Clinical Diagnosis by Laboratory Methods.* 15th ed. Philadelphia: Columbia Broadcasting System, W. B. Saunders Co., 1974.

Davis, B. D.; Dulbecco, R.; Eisen, H. N.; Ginsberg, H. S.; and Wood, Jr., W. B. *Microbiology.* 2nd ed. New York: Harper & Row Publications, Inc., Harper Medical Department, 1973.

Edeiken, J. *JAMA* 232 (1975):1366.

Hughes, H. E., and Dodds, T. C. *Handbook of Diagnostic Cytology.* New York: Longman, Inc., 1968.

Hurst, J. W., and Logue, R. B., eds. *The Heart.* 3rd ed. New York: McGraw-Hill Book Co., 1974.

Lehninger, A. *Biochemistry.* New York: Worth Publishers, Inc., 1970.

Lichtenstein, L. *Diseases of Bone & Joints.* 2nd ed. St. Louis: C. V. Mosby Co., 1975.

Robbins, S. L. *Pathologic Basis of Disease.* Philadelphia: Columbia Broadcasting System, W. B. Saunders Co., 1974.

Salter, R. B. *Textbook of Disorders & Injuries of the Musculoskeletal System.* Baltimore: Williams and Wilkins Co., 1970.

Stanbury, J. B.; Wyngaarten, J. B.; and Fredrickson, D. S. *The Metabolic Basis of Inherited Disease.* 3rd ed. New York: McGraw-Hill Book Co., 1972.

Strauss, M. B., and Welt, L. G. *Diseases of the Kidney.* 2nd ed. 2 vols. Waltham: Little, Brown & Co., 1971.

Takahashi, M. *Color Atlas of Cancer Cytology.* Philadelphia: J. B. Lippincott Co., 1971.

Williams, R. H., ed. *Textbook of Endocrinology.* 5th ed. Philadelphia: Columbia Broadcasting System, W. B. Saunders Co., 1974.

Williams, W. J.; Beutler, E.; Erslev, A. J.; and Rundles, R. W. *Hematology.* New York: McGraw-Hill Book Co., 1972.

Wintrobe, M. M.; Thorn, G. W.; Raymond, D. A.; Braunwald, E.; Isselbacher, K. J.; and Petersdorf, R. G., eds. *Harrison's Principles of Internal Medicine.* 7th rev. ed. New York: McGraw-Hill Book Co., Blakiston Publications, 1974.

Wintrobe, M. M.; Lee, G. R.; Boggs, D. R.; Bithell, T. C.; Athens, J. W.; and Foerster, J. *Clinical Hematology.* 7th ed. Philadelphia: Lea & Febiger, 1974.